THINNER AT LAST

STEVEN LAMM, M.D.,

AND GERALD SECOR COUZENS

A FIRESIDE BOOK

Published by Simon & Schuster

FIRESIDE
Rockefeller Center
1230 Avenue of the Americas
New York, NY 10020

First Fireside Edition 1997

FIRESIDE and colophon are registered trademarks
of Simon & Schuster Inc.

Designed by Irving Perkins Associates, Inc.

Manufactured in the United States of America

1   3   5   7   9   10   8   6   4   2
1   3   5   7   9   10   8   6   4   2 (Pbk)

Library of Congress Cataloging-in-Publication Data
Lamm, Steven.
Thinner at last / Steven Lamm and Gerald Secor Couzens.
p.   cm.
Includes bibliographical references and index.
1. Appetite depressants.   2. Reducing.   I. Couzens, Gerald Secor.
RM332.3.L36   1995
616.3'98061—dc20   95-24666
CIP
ISBN 0-684-81368-8
0-684-83035-3 (Pbk)

Obesity is a serious medical condition, and weight reduction requires careful consideration. The weight-loss treatment described in this book is intended to supplement, not replace, the medical advice of trained professionals. All matters regarding your health require medical supervision. Consult your physician before beginning a weight-loss program or adopting the medical suggestions in this book, as well as about any condition that may require diagnosis or medical attention.

The drugs described in this book have been approved by the FDA, and must be prescribed by a licensed physician. All prescription drugs have possible side effects. Consult a physician who is familiar with current medical literature and can explain possible side effects associated with drug therapy.

The authors and publishers disclaim any liability arising directly or indirectly from the use of this book.

Contents

Contents

Preface

No one can deny the ineffectiveness of the current approaches to weight loss. As one diet evolves and quickly fades—typically resulting in despair for the people who failed the diet—another springs up to take its place, replete with its own set of promises.

The good news is that *Thinner at Last* is not a diet book. While it details how you can successfully lose weight and keep it from coming back, it contains none of the common staples so typical of the weight-loss genre. I don't ask you to follow a "miracle" eating plan. Unlike other weight-loss books, *Thinner at Last* contains no gourmet recipes, nor are you asked to measure your food and calculate the caloric content of every morsel.

Instead, I challenge the conventional wisdom about weight loss and ask you—and your physician—to view excessive weight as a medical condition requiring medical attention. The opening chapters offer the most recent and comprehensive information on the pharmacological treatment of excessive weight. You will learn about the newest drugs available that help you lose weight, how they work, and why they keep the weight from coming back. In addition, there is a chapter devoted to low-fat eating and another which stresses the need for regular exercise.

I have successfully treated hundreds of patients with these medications and the many case histories throughout the book attest to the success of this approach. All names and identifying details of patients have been changed to respect their privacy.

This book is designed to guide and educate those who struggle with losing weight and have difficulty keeping the unwanted pounds from coming back. Throughout the book, I recommend that you consult your physician before taking any medication, undertaking nutritional changes, or starting an exercise program. While I hope this book will be of great use to you, it is not intended as a substitute for sound medical advice.

Since this book is about the latest scientific approach to weight loss, I have provided a special section in the book you can give to your physician that summarizes all of the key points. It's my hope that, working together with your physician, you will achieve your weight-loss goals and escape the diet merry-go-round forever.

A Note to the Reader of the Updated Edition

When I first started writing *Thinner at Last,* my weight-loss work was still considered controversial. Physicians, by and large, still had to be persuaded—oftentimes by their own patients—to use fenfluramine and phentermine. Many of my own patients were skeptical as well. That is, until they came to my office, began the fen-phen therapy, and soon discovered what they could only consider to be miraculous changes.

During the course of my therapeutic work with patients over the past four years, I have been aware of the new medication, dexfenfluramine. Although used extensively throughout the world for years, but not permissible in the United States, I knew it would be available at some point in this country. I also knew that, because of the specific nature of dexfenfluramine, the new drug could be used without any change in my treatment program. Now, with the approval of dexfenfluramine (trade name: Redux) by the Food and Drug Administration, in addition to prescribing fen-phen in combination to all of my patients, I now have the possibility of using yet another medication on a case-by-case basis.

Whether you, as a potential weight-loss patient, use the enormously successful fen-phen program, which I continue to prescribe in my practice, or the newer dexfenfluramine, all that you read in this book will apply equally to whatever medication your physician prescribes for you.

CHAPTER ONE

Following the Wrong Prescription

Dieting doesn't work. The approach is antiquated, ineffective, and not consistent with the scientific and medical knowledge of the past decade. Advice about weight loss—which relies on willpower, nagging, and deprivation—has resulted in despair, anxiety, and self-loathing. Just ask any of my patients. They have tried every "hot" weight-loss plan imaginable, whether it appeared in a best-selling book or was given to them in confidence by a friend who swore by it. My patients have sojourned at every major "fat farm" and health spa in the world. And although they've collectively lost tons of fat, slimmed down, and felt great for a while, as soon as they stopped dieting, they slowly put the weight back on. Plus, in most instances, a few extra pounds.

Statistics show that virtually everyone who diets will initially lose weight but eventually regain most or all of it. We all know this, but still the desire to lose that extra fat remains part of the American psyche, with half of the population—and as much as 70 percent of American women—currently restricting their food intake in an effort to become thinner.

Once I would have encouraged these people. I, too, believed that a combination of diet and exercise was the best way to "cure" an overweight condition. During the past decade of work with patients, however, I have come to a different conclusion. I have learned that obesity is a chronic medical condition that needs regular treatment and management for life. Telling individuals to eat less when they are overweight is equivalent to telling a person with asthma to stop wheezing. And just as a diabetic or hypertensive person can't be expected to control his or her ailment without a suitable diet and medical program, neither should an overweight person.

My change in thinking is due to the new research about obesity and the important medical information that has been made available to physicians that is based on metabolism, physiology, psychology, and genetics. We now know that overweight people are not to be blamed for their poundage simply because there isn't a liquid diet, exercise video, or fat-free cake that can negate their genetic makeup. Far from being a character flaw, recurrent overweight problems require a different form of treatment, and that treatment is what I will explain to you in this book. Programs such as mine, despite their safety and reliability, are just beginning to come into use. So, for most patients, it's surprising to learn that there is a new—and in many ways, easier—method of treating obesity. But once they become accustomed to the idea, and begin to follow my instructions, they find that it is really possible to master—forever—the weight-loss struggle.

One such patient is Anna Benedict. When she first came to see me, she was forty-two years old and weighed 210 pounds. Anna told me, in a low voice, that she had been "a fatty" all of her life. She said she never had many friends during her childhood in Manhattan. She was ridiculed and bullied every day in elementary school by cruel schoolmates who would cry out, "Make way for Tubby!" In high school, Anna had no dates, and most of the boys she came into contact with made rude remarks and ugly noises when she moved through the halls. When Anna was seventeen and 205 pounds, she got a prescription for diet pills (amphetamines) from her family doctor, and after six months of pill taking and following a 900-calorie diet, she shed 75 pounds. She stayed on the pills for eight years, maintaining her weight at 130 pounds, but at the same time suffering all the side effects of amphetamine abuse: insomnia, mood swings, edginess, and hair-trigger temper. Increasingly frightened by these effects, Anna stopped using the pills and slowly regained the weight she had fought so hard to keep off.

She then tried every weight-loss program she heard about: the Cambridge Diet, the Scarsdale Diet, the rice diet, Weight Watchers, and Optifast. She went to one Overeaters Anonymous meeting but left in despair before it was over because she didn't really think she was overeating. She took in only 1,100 calories a day, she was starving herself, and still she gained weight.

By the time Anna got to my office, she was desperate. Her eating habits and her weight gain simply didn't add up. She needed answers, yet she had almost given up hope of getting any. Still, like many overweight people, Anna was brave and determined to succeed.

It took Anna a while to understand the differences between

my treatment and those she had already experienced. She had to accept the idea that medication would play an important role in the program, but that the medication would not cause the unnerving side effects of amphetamines. In fact, depending on the person, it had few bothersome side effects, and these could easily be controlled. Although she was a little apprehensive at first, Anna found the program simple to follow and effective. It worked because it got to the heart of Anna's condition—a genetic imbalance that caused her to gain weight more easily than she should have.

Anna now weighs 145 pounds, has maintained that weight for over three years, and is off the medication. She is on her way to a master's degree in education, but most important, she is intimately involved in the management of her condition and at the first sign of an alarming weight increase—for whatever reason—she goes right back on medication under my supervision.

Anna is just one of hundreds of my patients who have succeeded in losing weight and keeping it off using this totally new approach. Before I go into the details of my program, you'll need to understand, if you're a frequent and failed dieter, how you got to where you are now, and why the old techniques you've employed are not solutions.

Are You Overweight?

To begin, let's look at whether you actually are overweight—or are instead chasing after the excessively slim ideal promulgated by the media. Unfortunately, most women measure themselves against fashion models, which is certainly unrealistic and even dangerous. The average woman is 5′3″ and weighs 144 pounds. Compare this to the average model, who is typically between 5′10″ and 6 feet and weighs between 115 and 120 pounds.

About one-third of all Americans are above their ideal weight as determined by standard tables, such as the Metropolitan Life Insurance tables of "ideal" weights. If you are 20 percent higher than the desirable weight for your particular height, you're considered obese. For instance, a 5′4″ woman who weighs more than 157 pounds is obese. So is a 6-foot man who weighs more than 200 pounds. But whether you are obese, moderately overweight, or somewhat overweight, you are probably not alone in wanting help.

Your Problem Is a National One

If obesity were viewed as tuberculosis or some other public health issue, you can be sure health officials would have declared a national epidemic a long time ago. They may do so soon, though, because Americans—who already lead the world in obesity rates—are getting even fatter. Recent statistics from the Centers for Disease Control and Prevention's National Center for Health Statistics indicate that 33 percent of American adults are overweight or obese, up from 25 percent in 1980. Moreover, the rise of obesity among teenagers—21 percent of all twelve- to nineteen-year-olds are overweight—is a frightening omen.

Besides the genetic basis for obesity (the *ob* gene), which has only recently been discovered by Jeffrey Friedman at The Rockefeller University, the weight increase can also be linked to the availability of high-fat foods and to physical inactivity. Never before in human existence has a group of people had to move their bodies so little. We use cars and rarely walk. We have elevators and escalators, so we no longer have to walk up flights of stairs. We ride on mowers, so we don't have to push a lawnmower around the yard. TV viewing, especially by adolescents, is at an all-time high. Thus, it's not surprising to learn that one-half of the U.S. population is relatively sedentary and 30 percent is almost totally sedentary.

Most Americans expend only one-fourth the calories burned by their ancestors in 1900. Whereas the old-timers had about 500 food items to choose from a century ago, we have more than 50,000 such items, and plenty of leisure time for eating.

The struggle to lose weight and keep it off is so pervasive that, according to the National Institute of Mental Health, 70 percent of young women between the ages of fourteen and twenty-one are on diets, a task most of them will continue throughout their adult lives. For some, this leads to eating disorders such as anorexia and bulimia. Desperate for solutions to their weight problems, they—and other dieters—go from physician to physician and then from program to program. But it has become increasingly evident that both the healing professions and the vast services that have grown up around dieting have generally failed to meet the needs of the overweight.

Where the Medical Profession Falls Short

Doctors are dedicated to helping people get better. But, unfortunately, they too often look at excessive weight as the cause of a problem, rather than a problem in itself. A person with chronic back pain, for example, may be told to "take off about 20 pounds," as if, for most people, that were easily done. And, once a physician has noted that a patient is overweight, there's a tendency to blame every medical complaint, whether a sore foot or a headache, on the extra pounds.

Even doctors who recommend diet and exercise often fail to be specific. "He told me to eat the right foods, but I didn't have the slightest idea what he meant," one patient said of his internist. Other doctors will hand a patient a pamphlet on exercise guidelines but not take the time to review its contents.

In short, many physicians are not tuned in to the difficulties of losing weight. They can make it sound too easy—when every overweight person knows that it's not—or they can treat the patient in a way that seems to be judgmental. Too often, a doctor can act as if an obese patient is weak-willed or lazy, even if he or she doesn't come right out and say so. "My doctor always made me feel like a naughty child," was the way one of my patients summed it up.

When patients feel this way, they inevitably turn to what has been termed the Diet Industry. Comprising health clubs, low-fat, low-calorie prepared food companies, diet book publishers, exercise videos, weight-loss seminars, and overweight support groups, it is a major business enterprise that, by some estimates, currently grosses between $30 billion and $50 billion annually.

Granted, the industry has met some of the needs of the overweight by creating the nonjudgmental, supportive environment not found in many doctors' offices. Certain groups have attempted to create nutritional programs that meet appropriate standards, while others offer behavior modification programs and exercise plans.

For the most part, however, these groups have failed to help people keep weight off because they lack a basic understanding of the genetic, physiologic, and metabolic aspects of weight management and of the neurochemicals that affect hunger and appetite. (An explanation of these factors, which is an important part of my program, will be detailed in the next two chapters.) Diet Industry groups also try to hide, for the most part, the sad truth about dieting, which is: In most cases, the effects do not last.

How Diets Go Wrong

You've probably discovered that losing weight is not the major problem—you may have done it countless times over the years. Keeping the weight off is the hardest part.

Evidence presented at a National Institutes of Health conference on obesity in 1992 showed that the average dieter in a commercial weight-loss program regained one-third to two-thirds of the lost weight within a year, and nearly all of it within five years. Ultimately, 90 percent of dieters regain all the weight they've lost.

Why?

When you diet, two critical physiological factors work against you. First, evidence suggests that the hypothalamus of the brain—although it is likely that other parts of the brain will be shown to be very important—works to maintain your current weight or *set point*. The brain guards against underconsumption (this is what dieting is), while offering only a weak defense against overconsumption. When you cut back on food, the brain signals a need for more. At the same time, it also lowers metabolism, so that the body stores more fat, making it harder for you to reach your dieting goals. In prehistory, our fat-storing ability was essential to survival. Today, of course, it is a liability.

The activity of the hypothalamus partly explains why it can be so difficult to take off 10 percent of your weight and keep it off. Once you lose 20 pounds, for example, your body becomes used to the restricted diet you've been following. If you increase your food intake—even though you eat less than before your diet—your body treats the increase as excess and you begin to gain weight.

The second critical factor that makes weight loss difficult has to do with your muscles. The muscles are like huge motors, constantly working. They consume large amounts of calories, even when you are at rest, and thus, actually help to keep weight off. However, if you go on a diet of less than 1,200 calories a day, your body, in an effort to conserve fat stores, will begin to break down your muscles for use as an energy source. As a result, you end up losing muscle tissue as well as fat. Your weight may drop, as measured on your bathroom scale, but you will actually be fatter because your percentage of body fat has increased in relation to muscle mass. With reduced muscle mass, your metabolism works even more slowly, sabotaging any weight-loss effort.

These factors explain why you set yourself up for weight regain when you artificially restrict calories. Although dieting may yield short-term windfalls, you're really only accumulating I.O.U.'s, which your body will eventually want paid back with interest.

If you've tried one diet after another, you've probably noticed that it took progressively longer each time to shed pounds. And once you stopped dieting, you gained them back more rapidly. Studies on rats subjected to repeated cycles of dieting and regaining weight have confirmed this, showing that with each successive cycle, weight regain occurs faster and weight loss takes longer.

The Psychological Dangers of Yo-Yo Dieting

A 1994 report by the National Institutes of Health associated weight cycling with a number of adverse psychological effects. These include depression and negative body image. Having your weight go up and down like a roller coaster also affects the way people interact with you, so poor personal relationships are not uncommon among yo-yo dieters. When you lose weight, people applaud. When you gain it back, they're disappointed, and you feel your self-esteem plummet.

Evelyn Harris, one of my patients, had a long history of yo-yo dieting. She had reached her "ideal" weight at least fifteen times, and then the unwanted pounds came back on. "When I first reach my goal, it's great," Evelyn told me. "I love having my family and friends comment on my appearance. I can't wait to get to the store and buy some new clothes. And my son always makes a big deal out of whistling when I go by."

But when Evelyn gained back the weight, the whistling stopped, and although her friends never said anything, she could silently feel their disapproval—or she thought she did. "It's like having a big hit in a movie, or something, and then falling flat on your face the next time out," Evelyn confided. "I always feel like a failure, and it's harder to start dieting again the next time."

But Evelyn, like many of my other patients who had been frustrated by the cycle of dieting, always did try again, even though, before she came to see me, she wasn't aware of how much the odds were stacked against her. She blamed her own "lack of willpower," which—as you'll learn later on—had absolutely nothing to do with her dieting failures.

Still, Evelyn kept trying, as you probably have, because she genuinely wanted to lose weight. And with good reason, since extra pounds contribute to high blood pressure, non-insulin-dependent diabetes, gout, osteoarthritis, gallbladder disease, coronary heart disease, and certain types of cancer.

Being overweight in a society where ideals of thinness are so heavily promoted by the media also carries a social stigma. Heavy people are often viewed as less competent, less attractive, and less likable. In one study involving college students who were asked to look at characteristics for suitable mates, embezzlers, cocaine users, and shoplifters were all rated as more suitable partners than the overweight. And in another study, small children looking at silhouettes of overweight kids described them as dirty, ugly, lazy, and dishonest.

I find that very often overweight people are too affected by such stereotypes or influenced by our unrealistic expectations of beauty, particularly for women. Nevertheless, the desire to lose weight is generally a good one and should be supported, once the person understands the physiological reasons for past failures and that he or she can benefit from trying something new.

Are You Ready for a New Approach to Weight Loss?

If you've tried unsuccessfully to lose weight without gaining it back, you've probably indulged in an orgy of complaints at the unfairness of it all. Sometimes your litany may sound, even to yourself, like self-pity, but actually, such remarks often point to a genetic component that's making weight loss impossible for you.

For example, a thirty-eight-year-old computer programmer told me that she faithfully observed the diet she had been given by a self-help group, and she showed me three weeks' worth of diaries that recorded every morsel she had taken in. Tossing the diaries on my desk, she lamented: "Life isn't fair. I eat a Spartan meal and remain at the same weight. My friends eat like lumberjacks and they still lose weight."

A forty-two-year-old advertising account executive went on a diet with her husband. Within two months, the husband was receiving compliments on his trimmer waistline, while the executive noticed only a slight improvement in her figure. She was furious. "I starve myself to lose two pounds in a few weeks," she complained, "and he drops ten with no problem. I get disgusted at my inability to do something that should be so simple. What's wrong with me?"

What was wrong for both of these people was the genetic and metabolic imbalance I mentioned earlier. For such patients—and I believe they constitute the majority of dieters—traditional approaches fail, not because the dieters lack willpower, but because of physiological reasons that are beyond their control. This is why something as "simple" as losing a few pounds can become a lifelong struggle.

If you, too, are blaming yourself, consider some of the statements you've been making to yourself. Do you ever say to yourself, I could lose weight if . . .

I didn't eat too much.

I didn't eat the wrong kinds of food.

I was able to exercise more.

I didn't have such a low metabolism.

I wasn't going through a stressful period at work.

I drank more water.

My bones and muscles weren't so heavy.

I could walk by a bakery without having to go in.

Everyone in my family weren't so big.

I didn't eat so much junk food.

I had better self-esteem.

I weighed myself more often.

I could stop eating when I'm depressed.

I didn't eat so quickly.

I didn't have to eat in restaurants all the time.

I didn't wake up in the morning dreaming of french toast.

I was normal.

I've heard all of these "ifs" and then some from my patients. Many expect me to chastise them for "rationalizing" when they should be dieting more. But I explain that such so-called rationalizations often mean that traditional approaches can't and won't work for them. Weight loss is a complex matter. They need to use an approach that can put an end—once and for all—to failures, complaints, and self-blame.

What My Method Is All About

I tell my patients that there is no medical condition as frustrating, mysterious, and difficult to treat as a chronic weight problem. One thing is clear, though: Human beings are far too complex to conform to an equation that says to weigh x pounds you must take away y calories.

Currently, nutrition and mental health experts are looking beyond calories and bathroom scales to examine a person's lifestyle, including attitudes, exercise habits, psychological health, and social support networks.

But the major solution—as researchers such as Jeffrey Friedman, Sarah Leibowitz, and Michael Weintraub have discovered in the past five years—centers on the physiologic and genetic link and the use of medication to achieve weight loss and maintain it. This is exciting news because it gives us direct insight into obesity as a medical issue for the very first time. We now know that the answer to long-term weight loss lies in a pharmacological approach, coupled with more familiar staples, such as proper nutrition and regular exercise.

In short, the basic focus has shifted to biology, chemistry, and genetic makeup—and that is how I now approach the treatment of obesity. I inform each patient that he or she must be prepared to do everything necessary to treat this ailment, a disease more resistant to successful therapies than many cancers.

Note my use of the word *treat*. My practice has taught me that obesity is not curable, but weight can be managed and maintained when medication is used. Once my patients realize that keeping the disease of obesity in ''remission'' involves constant vigilance and a combination of healthful eating and exercise, positive long-term results can be achieved.

My patients have learned to control their weight without feeling deprived, hungry, or locked into ineffective yo-yo cycles. They can make effective choices about exercise and eating. They feel ecstatic at finally getting control of their lives.

My approach is not a radical diet that relies on strange food combinations, powders, prepackaged diet foods, or liquid supplements. It includes a program of sensible eating, body-fat assessments, and regular sessions of aerobic exercise and resistance training. But as we shall see, it also centers on all-important new biological discoveries and the use of medication that has proven itself to be almost magical.

Clearly, we are at the outset of an exciting new era. Physicians like myself have finally been able to get weight management back into the medical realm where it belongs—and out of the hands of the Diet Industry. In the following chapters, you will see exactly how that was done and how you stand to benefit.

CHAPTER TWO

Solving the
Obesity Puzzle

I never set out to be a "diet" doctor or even to build a practice that had weight management as a major component. But, thinking back on it, my interest in obesity has been with me a long time. It dates back to my days as a student at New York University Medical Center, which is where I first noticed that there was something odd about the way the curriculum handled obesity.

My fellow students and I were taught that excess body weight was linked to a multitude of diseases that could eventually kill a person—hypertension, atherosclerosis, and diabetes, just to name a few. We learned that virtually every organ in the body is negatively affected by excess weight. Fatty livers, gallbladder problems, degenerative arthritis involving the weight-bearing joints of the hips and knees, hiatal hernia, chronic back problems—too much body fat was a culprit in every single one of them.

We were also taught about sleep apnea, a less common but certainly dangerous ailment linked with obesity. This potentially life-threatening disorder keeps you in a strange half-awake, half-asleep twilight zone. Besides leaving you perpetually drowsy by disrupting your sleep, apnea places a severe strain on your cardiovascular system and can lead to hypertension, nighttime heart attacks, cardiac arrhythmias, and stroke.

But even as we were instructed in the weight-disease connection, in practice, we focused only on treating the disease, not the underlying problem of weight. Obesity, though quite common in the patients we saw, was virtually invisible when we would-be doctors, under the guidance of our mentors, set about deciding on a course of treatment.

A patient who had a chronic back problem, for example, was referred to the physical therapist; a patient with hypertension was put on medication. Certainly there were special "diets," such as those required for diabetic patients, but these diets were usually the province of the nursing staff. It was the nurses and nutritionists who explained the diets to the patients, told them what food substitutions to make, and if they had time in their busy schedules, tried to motivate the patients to stick to the diets.

Weight problems were not medical problems, I observed. They were something to be handled, if at all, by some other type of health professional whose training was not as lofty as our own. I don't recall a single lecture by any of my professors that called for the management of obesity. Nor was there ever a discussion of nutrition or exercise. Unfortunately, although there have been a few changes, such gaps still exist today. A third-year medical student who recently came to observe me in my office explained that there had been no discussion in any of his classes about obesity, except from the standpoint of viewing it as a psychosocial disorder. So it's not surprising that many physicians aren't motivated to find the answers overweight people seek.

There are hopeful signs for change, at least from the younger set. My fifteen-year-old-daughter, Suzanne, has already had lengthy discussions in her high school science class about the genetic implications of obesity.

The Chronically Overweight: The Problem That Wasn't There

Green as I was in medical school, I remember having the sense that something was amiss. At every turn, I was taught to ask questions—about a patient with a heart condition, for example. Was his heart pumping blood efficiently? Were his kidneys excreting wastes as they should? Was there a bacterial agent or toxin at work? Did his mother, father, or grandparents have a similar ailment? Day after day, questions about each disease, common and rare, were "presented" to me by a senior physician. But when it came to obesity, the most pervasive metabolic disturbance in humans, there were no questions. Physiology, etiology, and genetics went out the window.

One night, during my internship, I watched a 300-pound man in the end stages of heart disease. He lay on the bed, totally colorless, hooked up to a variety of tubes, and getting oxygen through a mask. This patient, George Harlow, had undergone several hospitalizations during the previous months, and each time we experimented with different drugs. There was a genetic component to George's condition—his father had died from a similar disorder—and George had once told me sadly that he regretted having to "check out" so early. He was only forty years old and the father of two young children who came to visit him whenever they could beg permission to be allowed up on the floor. I could see how much he loved them, and I felt helpless because I didn't have all the tools I needed to help George. I didn't understand how to make it possible for him to control his weight.

At two o'clock in the morning, shortly before George died, the attending physician remarked that "his heredity was killing him." By that he meant that the substantial surgical and medical history that George had amassed by his fourth decade had finally gotten the better of him.

There wasn't a single entry on George's chart about his father's obesity. A chronic overweight condition was not a part of George's heredity as far as anyone was concerned.

No Real Answers

When I became a resident, and later on an assistant professor of medicine at NYU who taught residents, I continued to be intrigued by the obesity question. I kept up with the research, and I learned that there were plenty of studies showing that overweight people often tend to eat more—no surprise there —but nobody answered the basic questions: Why were some people hungrier than others? And why did most people who lost weight regain it so rapidly? These, I thought, were at the heart of the obesity puzzle.

Another mystery was why my profession was so unsympathetic toward overweight people. Being overweight, as I knew from my medical school experience, was looked upon as a character problem, while maintaining the "ideal" weight was a sign of willpower. This discrimination extended to the medical profession itself, with overweight medical or surgical residents often looked upon by their colleagues as lazy, slothful, and less "intense."

These issues were always in the back of my mind, although initially they didn't play such a large part in my practice. I am an internist, and I chose internal medicine because I wanted to treat the whole person. As my practice grew I realized the extent to which I was treating obesity-related problems. I was surprised when I discovered that approximately 30 to 40 percent of my patients were overweight to some degree and suffering the medical consequences. These included hypertension, diabetes, sleep apnea, arthritis, digestive ailments, coronary artery disease, and endocrine disorders.

What I Learned from My Patients

I was also surprised by the emotional impact that excess weight had on my patients' lives. At first, I didn't know much about this, because overweight people tend to keep their problems to themselves. In fact, in a doctor's office, they'll usually limit their remarks to the self-deprecating, such as, "I should be ashamed to get on the scale," because they hope to ward off criticism by attacking themselves first. My instinct was to never condemn patients whatever they told me about their lifestyles and eating habits. (Usually, overweight people have enough judgments made about them by family, friends, and even absolute strangers.)

These patients had been battered and they were fatigued. In addition to their physical ills, they suffered anxiety, frustration, and despair. Most important, however, was that they had lost hope of ever feeling "normal." This feeling was expressed by many of my patients. They wanted to be like everyone else—that is, someone who isn't plagued by food concerns, someone who eats when hungry and stops when full, someone whose weight will remain consistently in a healthier, lower range without total deprivation and misery.

Most of my patients had spent a lifetime trying to feel "normal" in relation to food and weight. Each time they succeeded on a new diet they were seized by the acute fear of regaining the lost weight. This was very often the trigger that set in motion a pattern of overeating in response to anxiety. Naturally, this led to a rapid weight gain and the self-fulfilling prophecy had been realized yet again.

Some patients talked about lifetimes filled with taunts, exclusion, and constant stares in public places. "I hate to walk down the aisle when I first get on an airplane," one man told me, "because I know everyone is praying I won't sit down next to them. Sometimes I wish I had enough money to pay for two seats, just so I wouldn't have to see those awful looks on their faces."

A woman executive in her mid-thirties described how she had closed the door of her office and simply sobbed after being turned down for a promotion that her co-workers agreed she deserved. "My boss never admitted it, but I know my weight had something to do with the decision. I was too embarrassed to even bring it up."

Perhaps the most heart-wrenching problems had to do with the effect that being overweight has on personal relationships.

I've even heard stories of divorce after one spouse was unable to comply with a demand to "knock off the weight," as if it were simply a matter of sloughing it off. It's amazing how many people blame themselves in these situations, especially if they've been trying to get thinner for some time. "I guess I'm just too stupid to ever lose weight," a printing contractor told me after his wife walked out on him. This from an accomplished, warm, and loving person who must have brought a great deal of tenderness to his marriage.

"You're not stupid," I assured him. "You have a health problem."

Even as I spoke, I was thinking about how such "health problems" could be permanently solved. This was my constant dilemma.

From the first moment I realized the extent of the obesity-related problems in my practice, I knew I couldn't simply tell people to cut back at mealtime or go for a bike ride in Central Park. That would be failing my patients as their primary-care physician.

My Search for Solutions

I thought I had an answer when I agreed to be the director of a liquid protein diet program in New York City. This very-low-calorie diet (VLCD) program had two major advantages: It produced quick results, which kept up the dieter's motivation, and it removed the dieter from solid food and everything associated with it, thus dramatically reducing the hunger level. It was, in other words, a completely controlled environment, rather like being in a space capsule. I saw hundreds of people lose tons of weight by following the VLCD plan. One patient took off 75 pounds in 120 days.

However, I eventually came to see that even with every possible psychological and physical support, an overwhelming number of those who lost enormous amounts of weight with liquid diets regained it, once they returned to the real world of three meals a day. My patient who had the 75-pound loss gained all of it back within two years.

VLCD programs failed to take into account what obesity really is: a chronic medical condition that resists dietary manipulation, however well prescribed. And, for me, there was always that critical question of hunger. Why were some people so hungry, so connected to a need for food, that they developed this chronic medical condition in the first place?

Even though I didn't have the answer at that time, I saw that there were no one-shot solutions. Overweight conditions needed to be managed through a variety of *systems,* as I like to call them, which are still a part of my program.

One system is eating, with which every reader of this book is probably all too familiar. I have always tried to personalize my dietary instructions to a patient's preferences and habits, but dieting is still boring and difficult. I spend considerable time talking with people about what they like and don't like to eat and what their lifestyle is all about. If someone travels a great deal, I urge them to avoid the high-fat foods they will encounter in restaurants, on airplanes, and while on the go. If someone is unable to cook for him- or herself, I again explain the need to restrict daily fat intake as much as possible and point out the nutritious ready-to-eat products that can be purchased from the supermarket. I explain how to balance sensible food consumption with erratic working hours. But it is still dieting, and until everything for me as a doctor changed, thanks to the availability of an amazing drug program, my systems alone were not the ultimate solution I sought.

The basic principle of my system of eating, no matter how individualized the format, is pretty much what you would expect: Food intake has to play a central role in weight loss and maintenance, and energy intake of less than 1,200 calories a day is not likely to be successful in the long run. How much you eat and what you eat is still a major determinant of body weight. You need to eat plenty of vegetables, fruits, grains, and beans, while cutting back on those fatty foods, such as potato chips, ice cream, cake, and red meat, which seem to spark our primitive hunger urges. These foods are particularly dangerous for people, like my patients, whose hunger levels are usually set on "high." I do not stress portion control because I don't believe this is physiologic. Rather, I try to help my patients develop systems of eating that ultimately result in reduced caloric intake without leaving them feeling deprived or hungry.

I try to individualize my exercise system as much as possible, too, with resistance training (such as exercising with hand weights) given as much emphasis as aerobic training. I make it very clear to each patient that if they are not prepared to exercise on a regular basis, they will not succeed in keeping their weight off. The first question I ask, since many overweight people are exercise-phobic, is: "What can you stand to do?" For most patients, the answer is "not much." So I get them to try walking or, depending on the person's medical condition, aerobic exercises, stretches, jogging, swimming, or resistance training.

Mechanical devices, such as a StairMaster or a cross-country ski machine, put very little stress on the joints and work, too, if they get used. Sometimes that's a big "if." One of my patients admitted having a ten-year-old stationary bike with an odometer reading of below 30 miles. "It's a wonderful place to hang my clothes," he joked, shortly before I convinced him to switch to daily walking.

I frequently perform fitness evaluations in my office with computerized equipment to help me come up with an appropriate system of exercise for my patients. After looking at their graphed charts together, we both have a very good idea about their current levels of strength and overall endurance and can base exercise strategies accordingly.

Another system is the use of behavioral modification techniques to change eating habits. Frequently, people turn to food as a balm to soothe nerves and numb painful feelings of loneliness, depression, and isolation. Behavior modification is a way of confronting and altering such self-defeating patterns. In a small number of cases, these techniques, as taught by professionals, did help in weight loss, but, in the end, did not produce long-lasting or permanent results.

I'll be much more specific about my systems—diet and exercise—later on. For now, I'll say only that when I first instituted them, years ago, they were moderately successful at best. Despite the individualized diet and exercise regimens, a significant number of patients, though able to lose weight, were unable to keep it off. For most, permanent weight loss turned out to be a nearly impossible struggle.

I was not any more successful than anyone else, and as a physician who demanded answers to the obesity puzzle, I found this demoralizing. I determined to scour the literature with renewed vigor. Somewhere there had to be an answer.

Unlocking the Puzzle at Last

I found the answer in May 1992 when I read a research paper published by Dr. Michael Weintraub, an associate professor at the University of Rochester School of Medicine and Dentistry in Rochester, New York. That article turned my world completely around. Today, I think of my weight loss practice as existing *before* and *after* Weintraub.

Before Weintraub, although I had crucial elements in hand, I had only pieces. After Weintraub, everything came together, and I was able to give my patients what they had always begged me for—the chance to feel and act as "normal" as other people when it comes to food. To demonstrate the remarkable effects of Weintraub's discovery, let me tell you how it totally altered the lives of two of my patients.

Marilyn Johnson was an attractive, successful woman by any standard, even before she began her weight-loss efforts. At forty-two, this mother of two was a high-profile lawyer as well as a major figure in the arts, working tirelessly as a fund-raiser for a large art museum. Along with her husband, André, who was also a lawyer, and a partner in one of New York's most prestigious firms, she appeared regularly at some of the city's toniest charity galas and cocktail parties.

Marilyn had the energy of three people. The fact that she was 35 pounds over her "ideal" weight didn't concern her in the least. In fact, she attributed her stamina, skin tone, and youthfulness to those extra pounds. She told me she felt it was better to have them as she entered middle age.

Marilyn was chic and extremely attractive in couture clothes chosen to express her sexuality. Here was a happy, well-adjusted woman, successful in her marriage and a powerhouse in her career. Weight was just not an issue. She enjoyed a good relationship with food and had never dealt with dieting, even as a concept.

In the first ten years that she was my patient, I had treated Marilyn for a variety of minor complaints. We discussed her weight only as a possible future medical issue. I had never suggested that her 30-plus extra pounds were something to be urgently concerned about until the day some routine tests came back with startling signals. Marilyn was now borderline hypertensive and showed signs of adult-onset diabetes.

My initial—and unsuccessful—approach to Marilyn's newly identified medical problems was the recommendation of a carefully tailored eating plan and regular sessions of aerobic exercise. Being the practical person she was, Marilyn understood what she was up against and took careful notes as I told her what strategies to follow.

It was a totally different—and by no means improved—Marilyn who came back to see me several months later. Increasingly alarmed by her medical condition, worried about her health, and now frustrated because her weight-loss effort was a dismal failure, she returned to my office in desperate straits for counseling. Angry and losing her self-confidence, she told me she was in a serious bind. The need to carefully watch everything she ate, cut back on all of her favorite foods, and monitor her weight was something so foreign to her that it had thrown her completely off balance.

Now, instead of living a successful and fulfilling life, she felt defeated and drained by the need to count calories and focus on what foods she could and could not eat. She found herself consciously thinking about food all of the time and aware, for the first time, that she had a subconscious food obsession. There were certain food items she routinely included in her daily menu and without them she started experiencing cravings so severe that they were interrupting her normally focused work sessions. This insight added to her increasing anxiety.

Marilyn discovered that the more she tried to lose weight, the more difficult it became. She'd lose 3 pounds, then gain them back almost overnight. For this high achiever, dieting marked the first time she had met personal failure, and she found it unacceptable. To try to make some progress, she began to skip meals, which left her hungry and tired most of the day. To keep up her stamina, she went from three cups of coffee a day to more than ten. But as the weeks passed and the pounds tenaciously stayed on, her frustration level started to build. She was no longer sleeping well, and she felt frazzled and irritable most of the time.

Marilyn's exercise program wasn't coming along as well as she thought it would, either. While she loved to dance, she found the step aerobics classes too strenuous and candidly admitted that she felt ill at ease with the younger, much thinner women at the gym.

I clearly saw that Marilyn's efforts were not only going nowhere, they were making her life miserable. After listening to her story—a story I had heard only too often—I told her there was another answer. I said she could lower her weight with medication, carefully explaining that the two drugs I wanted to prescribe for her were not like the amphetamine diet pills of the past. Far from being experimental, these particular medications had already been approved for the control of obesity by the Food and Drug Administration and had been available for several years. She hadn't heard of them before because they were not well understood by many physicians and were, thus, underprescribed. I explained to Marilyn that I used these daily medications on enough patients to know I was succeeding beyond my wildest expectations in helping them lose vast amounts of weight and keep it off.

Marilyn cross-examined me on the history of the medications, their potential side effects, if any, and the exact way they would work. She wanted to know why I hadn't prescribed them for her immediately, rather than putting her through what she called "the nightmare of dieting." I explained that, as with any other ailment, I begin with a conservative approach—in this case, food modification and exercise—and resort to medication when traditional methods fail. At the end of our conversation, she agreed to try the medications.

Marilyn was back to see me in a month—and there had been a remarkable transformation. She told me that, after two days of taking her medications, she had experienced an incredible change. For the first time, she was becoming aware of something she had always denied—the fact that food was an obsession.

She described to me a process through which she had begun to detach herself from food. She was able to step back and look at her eating habits in a more analytical way because she felt full throughout the day and was no longer hungry. She was eating less but enjoying it more. Gone were the midmorning and afternoon pick-me-up snacks—eating habits she'd developed in law school and never given a second thought to. At mealtime, her portions diminished as she desired less.

Within one month, Marilyn lost 12 pounds, but more importantly, she regained her sense of equilibrium, her vigor, and her confidence. "For the first time in my life, my mind is truly not on food," she told me.

What I saw in Marilyn—and what I have seen in so many of my other patients who take the medications I will shortly describe—was a return of hope in achieving her weight-loss goals, a freedom from the despair of dieting, and a belief that she could live a normal, healthy life.

I told Marilyn that I wanted her to continue with the medications and also to resume her exercising and make it part of her weekly schedule. Three months later, Marilyn had lost a total of 37 pounds. She was exercising three times a week by walking, swimming, and bicycling, activities she now found she loved to do. Most significantly for Marilyn, each of her alarming health risk factors dropped along with her weight. We had finally succeeded. The drugs had done their work, and a vital, attractive woman was a winner once again.

Another patient, Dominic Strassa, differed from Marilyn Johnson in that he had worried about his weight all of his life. As a youth growing up in a food-loving Italian-American family, he spent more time in his mother's aroma-filled kitchen than on the ball field. By the time Dominic reached high school, he tipped the scales at 200 pounds and was, unquestionably, the "fatty" of the freshman class.

Distressed by his rolling hips and disappearing waistline, Dominic tried and failed at one "crash" diet after another. Then a family friend told Dominic's parents about a local physician who could give him "miracle" pills to take off the weight. These, unfortunately, were amphetamine appetite suppressants.

Dominic went to the doctor's office but never actually got to see the doctor. Instead, he was ushered into a small room filled with a dozen overweight men and women sitting uncomfortably on folding metal chairs. The stark white walls had framed diplomas on them and the venetian blinds were pulled shut on the windows. Nobody spoke.

A tape-recorded message was soon heard from a large speaker mounted on the wall. Dominic guessed it was the voice of the doctor. He spoke for fifteen minutes about proper eating and the need to cut back on one's daily intake of food. The tape finally ended with the doctor raising his voice to admonish his listeners. "You're too heavy!" he said. "Now, go out and do something about it!"

The entire group of "heavy" patients then shuffled into the next room where a nurse handed everyone a little paper cup filled with green, yellow, and blue pills. Dominic was instructed to take six pills a day, along with two diuretics, and then return in a month. Exercise was never mentioned.

The pills kept Dominic from being hungry. He soon began to lose large amounts of weight, but he felt so keyed up that he was unable to sleep. His mouth was always dry, and he was constantly irritable, snapping at close friends and family members. Even though he quickly lost 20 pounds with the pills, the side effects were so frightening that Dominic stopped taking them, and the pounds came back on.

In college, Dominic joined a Weight Watchers group, where he carefully monitored everything he ate, and tried to suppress his always-present thoughts of food. He attended the meetings religiously, applauded those who succeeded in losing weight, enjoyed the applause that he himself received, but cringed as he observed that many members of the group seemed to be "returnees," beginning their efforts anew for the second, third, or fourth time.

After graduation from college, when he began working both a day and a night job, grabbing snacks when and where he could, Dominic's hard-won "ideal" weight slipped away. He followed a succession of diets, but he could never get the food cravings out of his mind, and time after time, those cravings defeated him.

At mid-life, Dominic underwent severe emotional stress. His wife of fifteen years died in an auto accident and, just a few months later, he was asked to take over as CEO of a start-up software company with sharklike competition.

When Dominic first came to see me, he was at his heaviest weight yet—240 pounds—and thoroughly discouraged by his inability to lose weight permanently. Like Marilyn, he had succeeded at just about everything he had ever set out to do. But weight loss, which he had been assured by everyone should be a manageable matter, completely stymied him.

I recommended a program of walking, jogging, and reduced-fat intake, but when Dominic returned a few months later, I could see that he found the program a real struggle. By watching what he ate and jogging every other day, he had initially reduced his weight by a few pounds. But then additional hours required at the office had forced him to stop jogging, and he fell into the habit of eating late at night when he returned to a house in which he acutely felt his wife's absence.

At this point, I told Dominic that I wanted to prescribe two medications for him, to be used in conjunction with his diet and exercise program. At the word *medications,* he protested, remembering the "miracle" pills that had sandbagged him in high school. I told him that these pills bore no resemblance to diet pills and worked in a totally different way. They were not, I assured him, likely to make him uncomfortable in any way at all. As I talked, I could see the doubt lingering on Dominic's face, but when I finished, he gave me his commitment to try what I had suggested.

Over the next few weeks, the change in Dominic was quite dramatic. As had happened to Marilyn, he noticed his food obsessions diminishing, then stopping altogether. Urges to find a seductive slice of pizza or a piece of Italian cheesecake no longer crept up on him late at night. For the first time, Dominic realized how pervasive these urges had been and how much they had been his master.

And as they disappeared, he began to savor foods that were not fattening but good for him in a way he never thought possible. Now it was relatively simple, and even exciting, to alter his eating habits, to have pasta, for example, with less cheese and more vegetables, to relish creating and eating a salad.

"I always thought I enjoyed food," Dominic told me. "But now, I'm really enjoying food for the first time. Best of all, it's not ruling me. I can decide how much I want to eat and not wish I had some more as soon as I'm finished." What Dominic was describing is the feeling of being full—a sensation with which he was just beginning to become acquainted.

Within five months, Dominic was close to his desired weight. He dropped down to 175 pounds. His percentage of body fat went from 29 percent to 16 percent. At forty-six, he looked and felt at least ten years younger.

Dominic Strassa and Marilyn Johnson are just two of the hundreds of my patients who have gone from being miserable and despairing to healthy and confident. They are, in Dominic's words, "new people." And now, let me explain what these medications are all about and how our understanding of weight control has been completely revolutionized.

CHAPTER THREE

Brainstorm in a Snowstorm

The question of whether overweight patients could or should be treated with medication was the focus of Dr. Michael Weintraub's thoughts one wintery night more than a decade ago as he sat in the crowded lounge of the Kansas City airport and waited for the snow to stop falling.

The storm, which had started the day before and dropped more than 15 inches overnight, had forced the cancellation of all flights. Weintraub, en route back to Rochester, New York, had brought along an attaché case of research papers but had never gotten around to reading them. Now, with the unexpected layover, he had run out of excuses.

Weintraub had the papers with him because a colleague on the faculty at the University of Rochester School of Medicine had long been stymied in his efforts to help his patients lose weight. The colleague had found that, although he could aid his patients in dropping pounds, he couldn't help them keep the weight off. In desperation, he turned to Weintraub, a clinical pharmacologist, and asked him to research the literature about the current state of appetite suppressants. He wanted Weintraub to deliver a definitive lecture on *anorectic* medications, as the medical literature calls these drugs, as part of a series of talks scheduled on obesity.

When his colleague, who was also a friend, first approached him, Weintraub was reluctant to take part in the series. But his friend kept pushing him, so he did what any good researcher would do: He got out every book and paper on the subject he could find at the medical library.

The reason for Weintraub's hesitation wasn't only a general lack of interest in the subject, as he had told his friend. He also doubted that there was any anorectic drug available which could work well for patients. And even if there were such a drug, physicians probably wouldn't want to prescribe it. That's because they tended to lump all appetite-suppressant drugs in the same category with amphetamines—drugs that were widely prescribed by physicians in the 1950s and 1960s. These drugs had such unpleasant and harmful side effects and had been so widely abused that no physician wanted to be associated with them.

Over the "Speed" Limit:
The Rush Stops

Appetite-suppressing drugs are nothing new to medicine. The amphetamine Benzedrine was first introduced more than a half century ago to treat obesity, followed a short time later by Dexedrine. Most physicians who work with the overweight have encountered people who tried these drugs at one point or other in their weight-loss odysseys and each had pretty much the same predictable reaction.

The experience of one of my patients, a woman in her early fifties, was fairly typical. "Sure the pill worked; it was 'speed,' " she told me. "I started taking amphetamines in college, just like a lot of my friends. I had put on fifteen pounds during my first semester and I panicked. I didn't know what to do. My roommate put on even more weight. But when she came back from winter break, she had a prescription for amphetamines she'd gotten from her mother's doctor. It wasn't too long before I started to take them too. And bam! The pounds melted away—but so did my mental health. I'm lucky I got through school without cracking up."

Although many people who used the "black beauties" and "yellow jackets" did lose weight, they paid a steep price, both mentally and physically. Shaky hands, irritability, heart palpitations, elevated blood pressure, sleepless nights, agitation—these were among the all-too-common side effects. Some patients became "speed junkies," going for days with little food or sleep. Others saw their professional and personal lives destroyed. Some even committed suicide. In the end, many dieters realized that a svelte silhouette was simply not worth the cost of being addicted to the drug, and they quit cold turkey.

Amphetamines are addictive, perhaps because of their effect on dopamine, one of the key neurotransmitters—chemicals that send messages to the nerve cells—released in the brain. Dopamine makes us feel good. Among others things, for example, it allows us to appreciate a sunny day and enjoy the smell of flowers. The brain guards its release very carefully and only allows it out of a brain cell for brief moments. Dopamine's job is to go from one brain cell and plug into keyholes called receptors on other cells. Once dopamine delivers its message, it backs out and is picked up quickly by transporters, to be stored safely for future use.

Normally, dopamine pulses on and off as needed and everything works fine. As a result of taking amphetamines, however, the brain is tricked into releasing too much dopamine, eventually becomes overstimulated by it, and dopamine is prevented from returning to its normal "off" position. This prolonged exposure that brain cells have to dopamine eventually leads to trouble. Amphetamines cause dopamine molecules to remain in the brain synapse, accumulating and continuing to reward the brain cells. With so much dopamine now available, it's believed that this activates the brain's pleasure centers, initially producing feelings of euphoria, characterized by heightened awareness, confidence, and renewed stamina. "Speed junkies," those habitual users of amphetamines, soon develop an unnatural appetite for the drug and become addicted. And when they don't get it, depression often sets in. To feel good again, another pill has to be taken. Ironically, while the amphetamines' effectiveness for weight loss winds down after just a few weeks of daily use, the addiction continues.

In the ensuing years, as amphetamines fell from favor, countless former addicts stepped forward out of their isolation and shame and told their stories. Kitty Dukakis, wife of the former governor of Massachusetts and 1988 presidential candidate, Michael Dukakis, is a classic example of someone who unwittingly got caught up in the nightmare of physician-prescribed amphetamine abuse. Although Dukakis caused quite a stir on the campaign trail when she announced that she had been hooked on amphetamines for twenty-six years, hers is not really an unusual case. In 1956, when she was nineteen, Dukakis's physician first prescribed Dexedrine to help her lose weight. The drug, a stimulant, decreased her appetite while speeding up her metabolism. She weighed 130 pounds at the time and wanted to lose only 10 or 15 pounds. This may not seem like much, but it ended up causing her a lifetime of grief because of the hopeless addiction that followed.

Dukakis did indeed succeed in losing 15 pounds over a three-month period, but her daily 5-milligram fix of Dexedrine eventually became more important to her than her weight or her well-being. Despite constantly feeling irritable, cranky, and extremely impatient, she could not quell her craving for the pills, which continued even after her weight stabilized. For many people, this physiological dependence on the drug takes over and continues indefinitely. In Dukakis's case, the consumption of 9,500 tablets in a twenty-six-year span confirms the familiar pattern.

Dukakis successfully hid her pill taking from her husband. She tried to stop using the pills many times, but to no avail. In the early 1980s, after finally admitting that she had a problem, she entered a thirty-day detoxification program. But being the junkie that she was, on the morning she flew off to Minnesota to begin treatment, she dutifully took her diet pill. Fortunately, it turned out that this would be her last.

By the time I was in medical school in the early 1970s, amphetamines were no longer prescribed for weight-loss programs. Nevertheless, doctors have long memories and many of them are reluctant to recommend diet pills of any sort, despite the clear pharmacological differences between the amphetamines and the new diet medications.

It is those newer medications, definitively unlike the old pills, that Michael Weintraub read about in the Kansas City airport. His trip delayed by the blizzard, and with no indication when his plane would take off, Weintraub was reviewing information on appetite suppressants when something caught his eye. It was a description of nonamphetamine diet pills. The two most widely used were fenfluramine and phentermine.

A New Generation of Diet Drugs

Both phentermine and fenfluramine were "mind" drugs. They affected the brain's neurotransmitters, but they worked along more direct pathways than the amphetamines.

Like amphetamines, phentermine enhanced levels of dopamine and another neurotransmitter, norepinephrine, making them more available to the brain's nerve cells and thereby affecting blood flow, heartbeat, movement, and stress reactivity. Phentermine caused people to eat more rapidly, but to eat less, without the significant side effects of amphetamines.

Fenfluramine acted on another neurotransmitter, serotonin. Serotonin is involved in controlling mood and is thought to play a large role in reducing the feelings of agitation and deprivation that we typically associate with hunger. Serotonin also controls how much we eat, as well as the body's desire for protein and carbohydrates.

Fenfluramine was the first drug on the market to trigger the release of serotonin from nerve endings and prevent its rapid reuptake—or reabsorption—by the brain. The higher levels of serotonin seem to reduce hunger substantially by causing the brain to send a message that the belly is full. As a result, a person who is taking the drug puts down his or her fork a lot sooner.

These drugs seemed to Weintraub to be truly remarkable—

just the type of medications his colleague had begged him to find. Particularly exciting was the evidence that appetite itself could be controlled by changes in the brain's chemistry.

The promise of each of those drugs was enticing. Yet phentermine and fenfluramine had shown limited effectiveness when used alone in obesity treatment and physicians had become disillusioned. Was there a way to make them more potent and, thereby, more effective? Weintraub was struck by an idea. Often in the treatment of hypertension and certain cancers, physicians prescribe "chemical cocktails." By using two or more drugs, some stronger but with powerful side effects, some milder but with fewer side effects, the negative aspects of the stronger drugs can be offset by the positive effects of the milder ones. The end result is a treatment package that works much better.

What would happen, Weintraub wondered, if phentermine and fenfluramine were given simultaneously? Each drug influenced a different chemical messenger system in the brain. Teamed up, would they develop new strength, diminish each other's adverse reactions, and enhance weight loss? Pharmacologically speaking, this was a likely possibility.

Weintraub believed there was sufficient reason to begin a patient trial of the combination of anorectic drugs. While phentermine and fenfluramine were not new, the notion of using them in tandem was. Weintraub also thought that long-term use of the drugs should be tested as well. In the past, they had been prescribed only for three-month periods, because that was the length of time that FDA studies of each drug had lasted. This may have been a reason why each of the drugs had been considered "inadequate." Nothing found by these studies, however, contraindicated long-term use.

If obesity was a chronic ailment, as Weintraub suspected, why stop the medications after three months? The ultimate aim was not just weight loss, but to prevent the weight from coming back. Weintraub was primed to find out if the drugs would achieve this goal. Soon after returning home to Rochester, he designed the first human trial using phentermine and fenfluramine together as long-term medications for obesity. As soon as he received funding from the National Heart, Lung, and Blood Institute, he launched an ambitious four-year study.

The First Two Years

Weintraub put ads in the Rochester-area newspapers and went on local radio shows to explain the project and call for volunteers. The results were overwhelming. More than 500 people responded.

Using various criteria, Weintraub created a sample of 121 subjects, one-third male and two-thirds female, ranging in age from eighteen to sixty. The participants were 30 to 80 percent above their ideal weights, as measured by the Metropolitan Life Insurance tables. Their average weight was 207 pounds, which was more than 50 percent above what they should have weighed.

None of the subjects had high blood pressure, diabetes, or any other chronic disease, and none was on a long-term medication. All were excited about the prospect of being in the study, and all but one stated that they had seriously tried to lose weight in the past.

When the study began, the participants were required to reduce their daily food intake to 1,200 calories. They weren't given a specific diet, but they were shown how to make low-fat food choices and substitutions, for example, low-fat milk over regular milk, and chicken instead of beef. The subjects were told not to skip breakfast, to eat all meals slowly, and to be mindful of portion size. They all agreed to exercise for at least thirty minutes, three times a week, by walking, bicycling, or swimming. And they were also instructed on how to modify their behavior in situations that involved eating. So the familiar elements of weight-loss programs were in place. And, for the first month and a half, only these techniques were used.

During the sixth week, half of the patients, randomly selected, were started on daily doses of 60 milligrams of fenfluramine and 15 milligrams of phentermine. The other subjects were given a placebo, an innocuous substance that has no effect but is used to determine whether the changes that take place during a study are due to the drug being tested or to psychological factors. Both sets of subjects, those on the drugs and those on placebo, also continued with diet, exercise, and behavioral change.

Weintraub carefully monitored the group that was taking the drugs. The most common side effects noted were dry mouth, trouble in falling asleep, and unusually vivid dreams. But, for most people, these side effects were not severe, and they usually diminished or vanished altogether after a few weeks. If they persisted, the person was taken off the medications.

Seven months into the study, the participants were weighed. To Weintraub's amazement, the weight of 80 percent of the people in the drug group had plummeted. They had lost three times as much weight as the placebo group, an average of 32 pounds compared with 10 pounds.

Elated, Weintraub proceeded to the second phase of his study. He put all of the participants on the drug combination. Then, from among the subjects who had been on the drugs for seven months, he randomly selected one group that would receive the drugs continuously over the next few weeks, and another that would be "pulsed," that is, take the drugs in an on-and-off sequence.

The pulsing was to test whether a series of "drug holidays" would affect the weight-loss process. They did. As soon as patients stopped the medications, the pounds crept back. When drugs were resumed, the weight came off again. This discovery bolstered Weintraub's theory that obesity was somehow related to the chemistry of the brain. The pills didn't "cure" in the same way that antibiotics cure infections. Instead, they seemed to work as asthma and blood pressure medications do, to correct permanent physiological imbalances. Obesity seemed to be, as Weintraub had suspected, a chronic condition that needed long-term treatment. The evidence was quite graphic.

The Findings Were Impressive

As the second half of the study began, Weintraub experimented with drug dosages. He found that although the original dose was sufficient to keep weight off for most participants, some did better when the dosage was elevated. Those subjects who had not lost more than 10 percent of their weight, for example, lost greater amounts when he raised the dosage of phentermine from 15 to 30 milligrams. So, by making adjustments in one component of the "chemical cocktail," Weintraub was able to increase its effectiveness for some people.

In the final phase of the study, Weintraub developed a protocol that would further test the efficacy of the drugs. He randomly removed some of the subjects from the drugs, put them on placebo, and tracked their progress. The results were poor. The placebo subjects not only stopped losing weight, they started gaining back the weight they had already lost.

Once again, the role of the drugs in weight loss appeared to be central. This was confirmed during the final seven months of the study. Now Weintraub gradually removed the remaining drug users from the medication, although exercise, diet, and behavior modification continued. What happened? Ninety percent of these people started to regain weight, and at a fairly rapid rate. By the time the study ended, almost all were as heavy as they had been four years earlier. Only a scant 10 percent succeeded in keeping the weight off.

When the study was published in May 1992, Weintraub's major findings were impressive: 80 percent of the participants who took the drugs for four years had lost an average of 34 pounds—16 percent of their body weight—and they were able to maintain the loss until the drugs were stopped. Compared with those on placebo, the subjects on the drugs felt less hungry, became full faster, and had decreased difficulty in sticking to the diet. Weintraub concluded that phentermine and fenfluramine, working in combination, helped to reset the body's weight-control mechanism so that lower weight could be maintained. It was like permanently setting a thermostat at the level where it could do the most good.

For the weight-loss field, with its long record of failure, Weintraub's results were truly amazing. The data on the success of commercial diets, jaw wiring, behavior modification, balloons inserted into the stomach, and other methods were simply dismal. With the publication of Weintraub's study, at last there was good news. For many doctors, this was monumentally important. But still, in some quarters, there was the inevitable resistance.

For example, some of Weintraub's study participants found that their own physicians doubted the efficacy of the drugs, and refused to prescribe them, even after seeing the evidence. Even today, many physicians continue to believe that overweight people have only to close their mouths or push away from the table to lose weight. (In a later chapter, I'll explain how to find the help you need if you think you could benefit from these drugs and I'll also provide an information sheet for your physician.)

Weintraub finds the current situation frustrating. "It's as if a doctor were to say, I don't think penicillin is an effective drug for a bacterial infection, so I won't prescribe it,' " he commented. "It's hard to believe that any doctor, knowing his or her patient is going to fail on diet and exercise alone, would refuse to help by prescribing something that will work."

Yet, this is too often the case, despite the clear-cut results of Weintraub's study and another that followed it in 1993. In similar research at the Veterans Affairs Medical Center in Hampton, Virginia—this time using a sample of 506 women and 57 men—stunning results were also achieved. After being on the phentermine-fenfluramine combination for nine months, participants lost an average of 37 pounds. Improvements in health due to weight loss were also noted. The blood pressure of 49 hypertensive patients dropped to normal, and the cholesterol of 24 participants with high levels reached acceptable levels. Elevated blood sugar, an indicator for diabetes, was lowered in several patients as well.

This second study, by the way, answered the objections of some critics that Weintraub's original study had included too small a sample. Now there was evidence that the drugs worked for substantial numbers of people.

Nevertheless, Weintraub emphasizes, the drugs must be part of a comprehensive weight-loss program, similar to the one he used, which includes behavior modification, decreased fat intake, and regular exercise. He favors such exercise enhancers as walking instead of driving to the store, parking a distance from the entrance, doing yard work, standing instead of sitting when talking on the telephone, and using the stairs at home and, where practicable, at work. Regular activity is an extremely important health message, not just for the overweight.

Weintraub's Discovery at Work

When I first read Dr. Weintraub's research in a journal called *Clinical Pharmacology and Therapeutics,* I felt as if a new day might have dawned at last. I went over the study at lunchtime, on a day when a patient with a particularly heartbreaking story had just walked out of my office.

This man, a thirty-six-year-old actor of some reputation, had battled a weight problem all his life and now found that it was interfering with his ability to get the parts he wanted. He had just been turned down for a major role in a "big" picture—and this was the break he had been waiting for. The reason given by the casting director: "You've gotten too chunky. We don't have time for you to get in shape."

Over the years, he had tried everything, including low-calorie diets, liquid diets, diet groups, consultations with top nutritionists, and a personal trainer coming to his home to help him exercise. Still, the insidious gain he called "my agent's worst nightmare" seemed to be marching relentlessly forward. It would be wonderful, I thought, to actually be able to offer hope to this patient—to finally have at my disposal a mechanism that would answer the unspoken plea of all my patients: "Doctor, make me thinner."

Starting with the actor, I began to put certain patients on the phentermine-fenfluramine combination, using dosages lower than the ones Weintraub had found effective, and then tailoring them individually. The results were truly amazing. The actor lost 45 pounds in nine months—and his agent quickly got him a plum role. And I saw other losses like these:

25 pounds in four months

30 pounds in six months

50 pounds in seven months

58 pounds in eight months

60 pounds in twelve months

I didn't need a calculator to figure out that the aggregate weight loss of my patients numbered in the thousands of pounds. Most important, though, the pounds stayed off—with continued medication.

Of course, not every story is exactly the same, and not every patient has been successful on the medication. But for most —and that means hundreds of patients—fenfluramine and phentermine have achieved remarkable results.

Dosages of fenfluramine and phentermine have to be monitored and modified by an alert physician, working closely with the patient, because they act on the delicate neurotransmitters of the brain. Their effectiveness demonstrates just how closely weight is linked to the chemistry of the brain and also to an individual's "genetic blueprint."

In order to understand these exciting new drugs, and their potential effect on your weight-loss efforts, you'll need to understand the brain's role in regulating appetite, which I'll explain next.

CHAPTER FOUR

The Brain, the Signal, and the Appetite

For years, researchers have sought the scientific reasons for obesity. Why does one person seem destined to be thin and another fat? What is the mechanism that makes some people constantly hungry and others satisfied with fewer calories?

For a long time, we looked to the environment for answers. Some cultures within our society, for example, place a great deal of emphasis on food and eating. It seemed reasonable to expect that a person raised in such an environment would be hungrier than a person brought up in an atmosphere where food is not so central. Another theory was that some people were more likely than others to turn to food for psychological reasons, such as a need for comfort.

Recent research has altered the perception that environment alone is the cause of obesity. Scientists now believe that just about everything related to obesity is caused by the messages our genes send to the brain via neuropeptides.

The genetic component of obesity has been demonstrated in several studies on identical twins who have exactly the same genes. In these studies, twins who were raised apart weighed more or less the same throughout their childhoods and adult lives. In reference to body weight, studies with adopted children suggest a very strong link to the biological parents, *not* the adoptive parents.

The genetically influenced brain chemistry of overweight people appears to signal the body, in an insistent manner from the fat cells, to keep on eating. In some cases, this craving— the *hunger impulse*—can be very graphic, particularly if the genetic signal is set off somewhat later in life.

Charlotte Sanders was never heavy as a child. When she graduated from college and married, Charlotte was 5′4″, weighed 116 pounds, and wore a size 6 dress. But shortly after her twenty-third birthday, she began to notice that she developed a ravenous appetite every month a few days before her menstrual period. She felt famished all the time, despite consuming vast amounts of food, and she would continue to feel hungry until a few days after her period.

It wasn't long before the extra pounds began to show, and the weight caused more problems in Charlotte's marriage, which was never very strong to begin with. Her husband, Bill, a generally undemonstrative man, now complained that he was embarrassed to be seen with her. His attitude added to Charlotte's stress, and she found herself giving in more and more to the hunger impulse.

Finally, she asked Bill to help her set up a training program to lose weight. He refused, saying that nobody had put a gun to her head and forced her to eat. "You made yourself a fat slob,'' he insisted. ''You're so large you should apply for state-hood.'' After that conversation, Charlotte couldn't stand to be near him anymore, and their sex life ended. Of course, the tensions in the marriage only made her want to eat more. Eventually, Charlotte and Bill were divorced, but the food cravings continued.

When she reached 220 pounds, Charlotte realized that she had come to a major turning point. No longer able to delude herself that she was simply pleasantly plump, she focused on what she found distressing about being overweight. She noticed, for example, that the man who worked at the fruit market no longer flirted with her. In department stores, it seemed to her that other women snickered when she tried on dresses. To avoid embarrassment, she asked her mother, an accomplished seamstress, to make her clothes, as she had when Charlotte was a child.

Charlotte also noticed that her friends related to her differently. Invitations to dinner dwindled. Some people stopped calling altogether. At work, her colleagues seemed too busy with one project or another to have lunch with her. Charlotte had never imagined that one day she would be so heavy and socially isolated. There were many times when she felt she might go mad from loneliness and shame. It all seemed like a horrible mistake. Deep inside, she saw herself as a thin person, kept prisoner in the body of a huge stranger.

Charlotte went to see a doctor who treated obesity and, for the first time, she heard about a possible medical explanation for her condition. She also heard about the amazing drugs phentermine and fenfluramine. For Charlotte, the effect of these drugs when she started to take them was dramatic. Within three days she felt as if a switch had been turned off in her brain. When her period approached, she no longer had that same insatiable hunger for fat and greasy foods. In addition, Charlotte became calmer. It was as if someone had finally cut the bonds that were holding her prisoner.

Within six months, she lost 44 pounds and believed that her life had been given back to her. But when she reached her goal weight, Charlotte's doctor refused to renew the prescription. He let her know that he didn't want her to use the drugs as a "crutch" and that it was now her responsibility to keep the weight from coming back. But Charlotte didn't think of phentermine and fenfluramine as a crutch. Instead, she saw them as the first medical treatment that worked—restoring her real self. She shared these thoughts with the physician but to no avail.

Charlotte felt totally betrayed by the first person who had ever really helped her. After seeing how well the medications worked, she couldn't believe that she had to be condemned to her former life. She went into what she called a "blue funk" and within months was back up to 231 pounds.

That's when Charlotte came to see me. I prescribed the same medications, but I told her that I believed her condition warranted their long-term use. Currently, Charlotte has slimmed down to 160 pounds and is on the way toward her goal of 130 pounds. "It's hard to explain," she says, "but now I eat what I want and stop when I feel full. It's as if my mind and my body are working together instead of fighting one another."

Our Actions and the Brain

Charlotte's experience with the hunger impulse demonstrates what so many of my patients have learned: The brain determines how much you eat. In this century, we are discovering more and more about the powers of this remarkable organ. Since ancient times, people have wanted to know what part of the body made it possible for us to think, breathe, blink, and carry out thousands of other functions. But the ancients credited other organs with orchestrating these things. The Egyptians, for example, believed it was the liver that controlled our actions. They thought so little of the brain that they threw it away when embalming their pharaohs. Since the brain served so little purpose in this life, they reasoned, what possible need could there be for it in the next?

In 40 B.C., the Greek physician Hippocrates, the "father of medicine," suggested that the brain was responsible for directing the body. It wasn't until 1860, however, that a serious scientific investigation of the brain was launched by a French physician, Paul Broca. Broca, an authority on aphasia, located the center for speech in the area of the brain that is today named for him.

After Broca, other researchers followed, gradually solving parts of the puzzle of how the brain mediates our daily actions. It's not surprising that the work is still going on. The brain is our most complicated organ, consisting of 10 billion to 50 billion neurons, or brain cells, over 100 billion supporting cells, and trillions of connections.

With the advent of molecular biology, neurochemistry, imaging technologies, and computer science, enormous strides have been made in uncovering the mysteries of the brain in the last two decades. There is still much more work to be done and, as our understanding of the intricate workings of this marvelous organ unfold, you can be sure solutions and improved treatments for some of our more vexing medical problems—including obesity—will be introduced.

The Brain Transmits and the Drugs Stop the Signal

The brain is divided into several divisions and subdivisions, each responsible for different activities. The lowest portion of the brain, the brain stem, which is relatively small, controls such basic functions as heart rate, breathing, sleeping, and eating.

Located above the brain stem, and accounting for two-thirds of the brain's size, are the two hemispheres of the cerebral cortex, the most recent part of the brain to evolve. The regions of the cortex control sight, hearing, smell, taste, touch, complex movement, comprehension of language, and the ability to think, plan, and imagine.

The brain is a gigantic communications network constantly sending messages to the rest of the body. The communicating is done by the neurons, or cells, of the brain. Each neuron receives messages from other neurons through a set of branches called dendrites. A neuron processes the information and then transmits messages to other neurons through a system of fibers called axons.

There is no direct contact between the dendrites of one neuron and the axons of another. Rather, the message is relayed over a tiny gap—the synapse—by means of neurotransmitters, which are chemical substances. Neurotransmitters are released at the end of the axon and bind to molecules, called receptors, on the surface of the dendrites of the adjacent neurons. When a neurotransmitter couples to a receptor, it's rather like turning the key in a car's ignition. The receptors link up with other molecules that extend through the cell membrane to the cell. Once the receptor activates these molecules, the mission of the neurotransmitter is complete, and it is either destroyed or taken back into the neuron that released it.

There are several types of neurotransmitters, but serotonin is currently thought to be of greatest importance to overweight people. Serotonin, which has a significant effect on our moods, is associated with such common disorders as obsessive-compulsive disorder, depression, and obesity. Because serotonin affects the brain's ability to process sensory information, low levels of this neurotransmitter can make it difficult to focus or to think clearly. Low levels can also make a person crave food all the time, even when there is no apparent need for hunger.

Dr. Barry Jacobs, director of the neuroscience program at Princeton University in Princeton, New Jersey, and his associate, Dr. Casimir Fornal, have been studying serotonin for more than a decade. They believe that both overeating and depression may stem from the same source—low levels of serotonin—and that these low levels are caused by a genetic "defect" of sorts, which I'll touch on later. The important thing to remember for now is that this defect cannot be cured, but it can be altered by drugs.

Almost all drugs that change the way the brain works do so by tinkering with neurotransmission. Some, like heroin, mimic the effects of a natural neurotransmitter. Others, like LSD, block receptors and prevent messages from getting through. The two drugs we're most concerned with, fenfluramine and phentermine, work in the following ways.

Fenfluramine interferes with the process by which neurotransmitters are taken back up by the neurons that release them. This increases the release of serotonin and raises its levels, thus relieving the urge to eat. (Prozac, by the way, a drug most often used for depression, also raises serotonin levels, so in some cases it is effective for weight loss as well.)

Phentermine interferes with the way that messages proceed from the surface receptors into the cell interior. It has no effect on serotonin, but by causing people to eat more rapidly and to eat less, it plays an important role in the "chemical cocktail" devised by Michael Weintraub.

When Weintraub combined fenfluramine, a neurotransmitter-affecting drug, with phentermine, a central nervous system stimulant that decreases appetite, he created a breakthrough. We now have the most promising approach we have ever had for treating obesity.

When Patients Ask for the Drugs

Not everyone who comes to see me is a good candidate for appetite-suppressant medication, and I will not prescribe it simply because I am asked to do so. What counts very strongly is the person's commitment to treating his or her condition and to following all the steps necessary for success. There is no one type of life history that makes one an appropriate candidate for the drugs. I remember two patients who battled their weight problems in quite different ways yet both, I decided, would do well on phentermine and fenfluramine.

Frances Jefferson, a forty-one-year-old financial manager, was almost killed by obesity. When I first saw her in the summer of 1988, she was lying in a hospital bed. At 209 pounds, Frances was so desperate to lose weight that she had been consuming diuretics and laxatives in massive doses. These drugs had stripped her system of electrolytes and brought on cardiac arrhythmia. Her vital signs were so shaky that the attending physician didn't know whether he could stabilize her.

I didn't get to talk much with Frances that day, but later on, when she was well enough to come to my office, I heard about the long struggle that brought her to what could have been her deathbed. From the time Frances was in the eighth grade and weighed 205 pounds, she had suffered taunts about her weight. Nevertheless, despite her weight and her family's financial problems, Frances managed to work her way through college and graduate school. A few years later, she assumed complete support of her aging parents.

Although Frances was highly skilled at her job, she began to see that her appearance was an unspoken strike against her. For business, she had to attend many social functions, and the pressure to get her weight down became a constant source of stress. After she was passed over for several promotions, she began taking the diuretics and laxatives that eventually landed her in the hospital.

"I have a lot of responsibilities. I couldn't risk losing my job," Frances told me. "I had to get healthy by doing something about my weight." At this point, of course, Frances realized that the way she had been trying to lose weight was anything but healthy. Never again, she promised me—and herself—would she use diuretics and laxatives in this manner. She had heard about fenfluramine and phentermine. Would I prescribe them?

Another patient who asked that question was Harvey Brenner, a thirty-seven-year-old policeman with four things in common with Frances: a weight of over 200 pounds, constant urges to eat dating back to childhood, a good work record, and performance evaluations calling for "improvement" in appearance.

"My chief said it was embarrassing for a cop to be fat," Harvey told me, "and dangerous, too. Anyway, I feel like I'm giving the department a bad name. I seem to keep on gaining weight no matter what I do."

Harvey was what I call a serious dieter. He read diet books, counted calories, and measured portions, yet when he least expected it he would find the food urges overwhelming and yield to them. He was always certain that his latest diet would start to work "tomorrow." Yet, despite what he read in the books, no diet ever "tamped down" his appetite. By the time Harvey came to see me, he realized that he had to go beyond diet, and he told me that he was ready to commit to any program I might suggest.

Psychologically, both Harvey and Frances were good candidates for fenfluramine and phentermine because they were highly motivated individuals who had demonstrated the ability to work steadily toward achieving goals. Even Frances's misguided weight-loss attempts showed a high level of dedication.

First Steps

When I first see patients like Frances and Harvey, I take a complete medical history to determine whether a genetic predisposition toward obesity exists. I note whether their mothers or fathers were also overweight and if they themselves had weight problems as adolescents. I also ask which diet and exercise programs they have tried in the past and why these may have failed.

I ask my patients if they have any medical disorders, such as diabetes, arthritis, hypothyroidism, hypertension, gout, or sleep apnea, that may be affected by the excessive weight. If they do, I explain that I will both treat the disorder and the underlying condition, which is obesity. I perform a complete workup, including blood tests, an EKG (electrocardiogram), a stress test, if indicated, a body fat percentage assessment, and a comprehensive physical examination.

I tell my patients that obesity is an ailment that requires a lifetime of treatment. No matter how much weight they lose, they will still have the underlying ailment. But by working in partnership with me, they can expect dramatic changes that will eventually end in success. They will see their weight drop, then stabilize, before dropping again. Their weight may go up at some point, but if they continue to follow the program, they will again start to lose weight.

Treatment for obesity, I stress, is not a matter of a straight line or of following one recipe. Rather, adjustments will be made in eating habits, exercise, and drug therapy. What the patient must do is see me regularly, so that his or her program can be fine-tuned as needed.

I assure my patients that I will never blame them for gaining weight at any point, but I do get upset if they don't return to me for effective treatment. Since their condition is physiologic, genetic, and chronic, the important thing is to keep working at it and not to give up. The goal I establish with patients is usually a 15- to 20-percent loss of body weight over the next few months. In addition to cosmetic changes, this loss will also have great impact on their health.

Typically, I prescribe 15 milligrams of phentermine once a day, the lowest dose available. For most people, the drug is optimally effective at this dosage. I find that only a few patients need to take 30 milligrams. As with all medications, phentermine can produce side effects. Dry mouth is a common complaint. Other effects include mild insomnia, sleeplessness, or headache. The unpleasant side effects, as I noted earlier, usually lessen and disappear over time. Phentermine can also have a mild stimulant effect, which most people don't find to be at all unpleasant. I usually suggest, though, that phentermine be taken before 11 A.M., so that its stimulant effects will have worn off by bedtime.

I prescribe fenfluramine in dosages ranging from 20 to 60 milligrams. Here again, I prefer using the lowest dose that can be effective. Fenfluramine has no stimulant activity. If anything, it may make a person feel drowsy, but when taken in combination with phentermine, the drowsiness is offset by phentermine's stimulant effect. Other side effects of fenfluramine include nausea and diarrhea in the early phase of treatment, but with the low doses I prescribe, these effects typically do not appear.

Some people are reluctant to use the drugs at all, usually because they fear side effects. I try to explain that no drug that has ever been prescribed is totally free of side effects. Even commonly used drugs, such as antihistamines, which most of us consider "safe," produce side effects.

When we discuss the health risks posed by obesity, it generally becomes apparent that they are far greater than the dangers posed by the drugs. The percentage of people who experience serious side effects from fenfluramine, for example, is quite small, while being overweight greatly increases the risk of heart attack, diabetes, hypertension, and a host of other disorders.

If there is still hesitation, and I feel drug use is necessary, I try to get the person to try at least one drug. For someone who is somewhat depressed and lethargic, I generally recommend phentermine, since it may help to increase activity level. If the problem is the opposite—agitation and jitteriness—I recommend fenfluramine because of its sedating effect.

With all my patients, I stress that one person's nervous system may be more sensitive to a specific drug than another's and that drugs affect each of us individually, sometimes in unexpected ways. A medication that's intended for sedation, for example, may trigger agitation in a small group of users. The key point, I explain, is to recognize side effects, particularly uncommon side effects, and communicate them to me immediately so that I can make adjustments, if needed.

For most people, though, there are no unusual or serious side effects. And generally, as patients become physiologically adjusted to the drugs, concerns about side effects diminish. Many patients, like Charlotte Sanders, notice that their minds and bodies seem to be working together for the first time, and they come to feel secure about the drug use.

Follow the Prescription

Another subject I discuss with patients is the importance of taking the drugs every day as scheduled, preferably at the same time, so that remembering is easier. People who are already on several other medications need to be especially careful not to overlook their doses of fenfluramine and phentermine. Sometimes it can help to keep all medications in one place and to maintain a check-off list of which drug was taken and when.

All too frequently, life's pressures make it hard to maintain regular drug use. Marital problems, difficulties with the children, upheavals at work—when these problems occur, patients often feel they cannot be bothered with taking their pills. Losing weight either drops down on their list of priorities or vanishes all together.

One of my patients, Linda Norman, a buyer for a large discount store chain, had to make frequent decisions about whether to purchase items being remaindered by wholesalers. If she made a successful purchase and the products sold well, Linda felt pretty good and remembered to take her pills. If she made a poor purchase and the items sat on the shelves, Linda felt rotten, worried about losing her job, and forgot about her pills.

I told Linda that she needed to add a reminder to take the drugs to her electronic organizer. These drugs, I stress with my patients, are just as important as any business or personal matters they need to take care of. Each person I treat has his or her distinct ideas, developed from years of battling excess weight. These ideas, some of them good, others off the mark, can serve to disrupt compliance.

One problem is a phenomenon I've also noticed in other patients with chronic illness. As the ailment comes under control with medication, some people begin to think they have been cured. Often, they stop using the drug in order to test whether they still have the underlying disease. For example, I treat diabetics who cease taking their insulin and asthmatics who try to get by without their inhalers. When this happens with my overweight patients, I remind them again that their problem is chronic and that the drugs are part of a permanent weight-control solution. I try to give this warning the minute I notice drug use slacking off, before the pounds begin to come back on and they have to play "catch up" to get them off again.

Finally, success itself can sabotage compliance. I don't know why this happens, but sometimes a patient who has been losing weight and tolerating the medications well suddenly stops taking the drugs, practicing good nutrition, or doing exercise. I make it a point to tell my patients that this might happen. If it does, they must be sure to come to see me, no matter how embarrassed they are about the amount of regained weight. In our relationship, I say, there is no room for self-recrimination because it leads to shame, separation from the physician, and another demoralizing defeat in the struggle against excess weight.

The Safety of Fenfluramine

Since I've been prescribing phentermine and fenfluramine for my patients, I, of course, keep up with current research about these drugs. I have been aware of a drug called dexfenfluramine, closely related to fenfluramine in chemical structure, which has been used for years in Europe. This medication has twice the anorectic potency of fenfluramine, and although it is currently under review by the FDA, dexfenfluramine has yet to be approved for use in the United States.

In 1994, dexfenfluramine received quite a bit of attention. Dr. George Ricaurte and his associates at Johns Hopkins University in Baltimore published a study indicating that high doses produced brain damage in squirrel monkeys months after use had stopped. A short while later, a second study, conducted on mice by the Environmental Protection Agency, refuted the results of the Hopkins study. Dr. James O'Callahan, who performed the research, stated that, "We noted no neurotoxic effect."

Many of my patients contacted me after hearing about these two findings. I explained that some of the most commonly used medications in use today have been associated with serious, and sometimes fatal, side effects. Fortunately, this occurs very rarely. Serious side effects have been reported very infrequently with fenfluramine or with dexfenfluramine. In addition, after rigorous testing, fenfluramine has been approved for use by the FDA. To date, there has been nothing to indicate fenfluramine's use should be halted. On the contrary, the use of medication in the management of obesity is here to stay, and we physicians look forward to the next generation of new and improved drugs which will inevitably be developed (see Chapter 11).

For the present, I have confidence in Dr. Weintraub's drug combination and the wonderful things it can do for people. For many patients, these drugs can bring about a complete transformation in their lives or, as one woman put it, "They make me the me I should have been." Because so many overweight people pray for such a transformation, let's examine closely how the process takes place.

CHAPTER FIVE

The Moment of Transformation

"I've gone from frustration to inspiration, from despair to hope."

"I feel as if I've been reborn."

"I'm a totally new person."

"My family thinks I'm someone else."

These are some of the comments I typically hear from patients when they start to lose weight on phentermine and fenfluramine.

For people with a long, frustrating history of diet failure, these changes are truly remarkable, encompassing not only the physical but the spiritual as well. For the first time in their lives, patients will report feeling peaceful, happy, and optimistic about their work and personal relationships.

This is not to say that the drug combination is a "magic bullet." In weight loss, there is no such thing, only commitment and hard work. But the medications, by correcting imbalances and opening up the possibility of success, can generate a process of emotional transformation.

There are a number of steps in the process, and they're not the same for everybody. For some people, it's a fairly simple matter to adjust psychologically to using the medications and enjoying the results they produce. Other people need to counter various forms of resistance before feeling comfortable. For such patients, there is usually an anxiety that must be overcome before the process of transformation can begin. Let's look at the stories of two patients.

Medication Resistance

Like most of my patients, Jay Levin had a history of weight problems dating back to childhood. When he first came to see me, complaining of severe heel pain that made it difficult for him to walk, he weighed 300 pounds. Jay was a large man— and his bulk filled my doorway. I knew even before examining him that his weight had to have something to do with his pain, yet I concentrated on the problem he presented to me.

After a brief talk in which I recommended better-fitting shoes, Jay brought up wanting to "do something" about his weight. This was an effort he had made once in the past, he said, but without success. At thirty-one, Jay was an established inventor and entrepreneur, the developer of a children's toy that had swept the market one Christmas and now remained a staple of the toy industry. His company had grown from a one-man operation to employing a hundred people, including a staff of designers who worked under Jay's personal supervision. "I have to be there all the time or things don't come out right," he told me, explaining that the whole company would fall apart if he didn't remain "at the helm."

Jay's earlier effort at weight loss involved going to Weight Watchers, at his wife's urging. But even though he thought the diet was basically "sound," he had trouble listening to "silly" lectures and being weighed in every week. His wife's efforts to cook low-fat, nutritious meals were undermined. Jay resented her help as well as the help from his Weight Watchers group, which he saw as controlling and confining. "The whole thing made me feel like Dagwood," he said.

When I told Jay that I thought he was a good candidate for phentermine and fenfluramine, he hesitated, saying he would mull it over. "I think I can take care of this myself," he said, "without drugs." A few months later, he was back with more foot problems and additional poundage. We discussed the medications in greater detail. Jay reported, with some concern that his sister-in-law, a pediatrician, had advised, "You're in good health. Why screw up your body by taking pills?"

I pointed out to Jay that the health risks he faced from obesity were far more serious than any small risks the drugs might pose. He was already showing signs of borderline hypertension, and I was certain that if he continued on his present course, other problems would emerge.

"Give me the prescription," Jay said wearily.

Four weeks later, he returned for a follow-up visit looking rather shamefaced. Though he'd filled the prescription, the demands of work were such that he wasn't able to risk not "feeling well" as a result of the pills. Meanwhile, his wife was pushing him to begin, and he felt he was getting into another "Dagwood" situation.

I realized that Jay's fears, combined with his strong need to be in control, were interfering with his acceptance of the medications. He viewed them as a threat to his ability to stay "at the helm," which was the major motivating factor in his life.

I gave Jay a copy of Dr. Michael Weintraub's study to reassure him about the safety of the drugs, and I explained that by using them, he would not be relinquishing control but correcting a genetic imbalance. I asked whether, as an inventor, he would ever turn his back on a helpful discovery. The medications were simply that—an important new weapon in the weight-control arsenal. There was no danger of their turning him into a Dagwood.

This conversation, and several others like it, eventually enabled Jay to begin the medications. I started him at doses lower than the usual regimen, and gradually increased them. Within months, Jay had lost 30 pounds, lowered his blood pressure, and definitely improved his marital life. As for the medications, whenever we talk about them today, he can't remember what his concerns were all about.

Side-Effect Anxiety

Angela Baldridge, a fifty-two-year-old secretary, was ready to try something new to lose weight. She was getting older, she told me at our first meeting, and felt she was running out of time to do anything to improve her appearance and diminishing health. If these medications really worked, she wanted them. "Will you help me?" she asked.

I thought that Angela was a good candidate for the drugs. But I also noticed that she was very eager to begin using them. Sometimes when people are that anxious to get started, they don't listen closely when I explain the side effects they may experience in the first few weeks.

A week after I put Angela on the drug combination, she telephoned. She had already dropped 5 pounds, she said, and was no longer feeling ravenously hungry. In fact, she was finding it easy to cut back on certain types of food, as I had advised her to do. Despite these accomplishments, there was a nervous edge to Angela's voice. When I commented on this, she said: "Well, I'm feeling a bit jittery during the day. And when I talk, it's as if my mouth were stuffed with cotton. I know it doesn't sound that way, but that's how I feel." Angela went on to say that although she was thrilled with the weight loss, she thought she should stop taking the drugs and stick to eating modifications and exercise.

I explained to Angela that dry mouth and slight jitteriness were among the most common side effects of phentermine and that these usually cleared up within weeks. I urged her to bear with them and to continue with the medications. I also advised her to adapt to the side effects until they disappeared by making temporary changes in her routine. Perhaps she could keep a bottle of water at her desk and take drinks on a regular basis until her dry mouth cleared up. Perhaps she could avoid social situations, such as the dinner engagement she had scheduled with a contentious sister-in-law, until her jitteriness passed. The trick, I explained, was to do things that would enable her to stick with the medications until she reached the comfort plateau which, I assured her, would happen soon.

I told Angela to check in with me by phone over the next few weeks. I knew she needed the reassurance that I would be monitoring her safety. I don't mind how often patients call me. It's when they don't call that I mind because I fear they may have given up.

A month later, when Angela came to my office for a follow-up, I realized that our frequent chats had paid off. The side effects had completely cleared up and she was ecstatic. She was beginning to feel, she said, "like a totally different person, someone who's really on top of things."

Angela Baldridge had begun the process of transformation, a process I usually describe, in terms of my patients, as massive gains in confidence when hope replaces despair. These gains take place because the drugs, in addition to correcting chemical imbalances, serve as a catalyst that makes it easier, and even pleasurable, to adopt new eating habits and exercise patterns. Everything—medications, nutrition, exercise—comes together and reinforces the effectiveness of the process. Suddenly, the world changes, and the patient realizes that this time, with this method, it's going to be possible to win.

The Confidence to Eat Without Fear

Claude Kostner was a chef in one of New York's finest restaurants and the winner of several international awards. A darling of the critics, scarcely an article on food appeared without some mention of his name, which was synonymous with haute cuisine. Cooking was Claude's profession, his passion, and his undoing. "I'm like an alcoholic when it comes to food," he told me. "I can't resist it."

For a man who couldn't resist, the restaurant kitchen was a minefield. Here Claude was surrounded by every variety of food, including pastries, which he couldn't help "tasting" as they came out of the oven. Sometimes, he confessed, sheets of cookies disappeared. For years, Claude's one defense against rapid weight gain had been smoking. Cigarettes curbed his appetite somewhat, but after his father, a lifelong smoker, died of emphysema, Claude decided to quit the habit cold turkey.

He came to see me, he said, "after I realized that I had traded one health hazard for another." Although he could stop smoking easily enough, he just couldn't stop his compulsive eating. At 220 pounds, Claude's health certainly was precarious. Given his build, his ideal weight was around 150. So I was not surprised when my medical evaluation revealed signs of incipient diabetes and circulatory insufficiency. When I gave him the news, Claude looked at me sadly. "I was afraid of something like that," he said.

Claude was only forty-four years old and the recent death of his father had frightened him. He definitely did not want to die before his time, he told me emphatically. If it was a choice between his health and his profession, he was ready to give up his profession. "I've got enough money to get out of the business and retire right now," he said, "but . . ." His voice trailed off. I recognized Claude's terrible sadness at the idea of being without the work he loved. Before I had a chance to say anything, he began castigating himself for his inability to curb his eating. "I'm such a fool," he said.

The cravings could be corrected, I told him, by the use of two drugs, phentermine and fenfluramine. These drugs would also make it easier for him to alter his eating choices and to take up exercise, which Claude had told me he loathed. His usual mode of getting to the restaurant, which was less than a mile away from his home, was by cab.

The notion of a genetic link opened Claude's eyes. It explained why there was so much obesity in his family and also why many other chefs had no trouble walking away from food. "Some of them are as skinny as sticks," he told me, as if that was a reflection on his own willpower.

I told Claude that given his history, he might have to take the medications for the rest of his life, but his life, I believed, would greatly change for the better. Given his health profile, I considered this a fair exchange.

Within two days of starting the drugs, Claude began to notice improvements. When he had to taste a dish, for example, he was satisfied with a forkful instead of an entire plate. When he ate dinner with the staff before the restaurant opened, he only wanted half of his usual portions.

But even as the weight came off, Claude felt uneasy. Would the changes be permanent? In the past, when he had managed for a while to control his food urges, they returned with a vengeance and he found himself eating more than ever. Surely that would happen now.

It didn't. Week after week, the obsessive thoughts of eating evaporated, and Claude was able to concentrate on the aspect of his work he had been neglecting—the creation of new dishes. For some time, he had been almost afraid to be alone in the kitchen for fear of giving in to food impulses. Now he found that he could conduct experiments and remain totally focused on his task, even throwing out dishes that didn't come up to standard instead of nibbling at them. Gone, too, was that sudden need to open one of the stainless steel refrigerators and find something to soothe a hunger pang. The link between working with food and eating it was broken.

Claude experienced an incredible sense of freedom. He knew that it didn't matter whether he was in the restaurant or on his sailboat—he had gained the ability to control what he ate. Professionally, Claude has gone from one triumph to another, and the pictures in the press reflect his substantial weight loss. Now he is described as slim. But there's one triumph that only insiders know about: The chef is no longer the victim of his own cooking. Thanks to the medications, he has perfect confidence in his ability to be safe from the impulse to eat.

The Confidence to Emerge from the Cocoon

When Elizabeth Weston, a librarian for a pharmaceutical firm, came to see me three years ago, she was a woman ravaged by three ailments: arthritis, obesity, and loneliness. Excessive weight and constant pain had left her physically enfeebled and socially isolated.

Still, Elizabeth's sad condition didn't keep people she hardly knew from lecturing her. One day, a young man with a bad stutter who had just started working for the company, told her, "Aren't you ashamed to be so fat? Everyone knows you must have big psychological problems."

That remark demoralized Elizabeth, but it gave her the push she needed to *do* something. She searched the library's database, discovered my name in an article on weight loss, and decided to seek my help. As I talked with Elizabeth, I realized how much sorrow she had experienced in her forty-nine years.

When she was eleven, her father died of alcoholism and her

mother went to work in the small town's only factory, leaving Elizabeth to care for her three younger sisters after school. Elizabeth remembered preparing white bread with mayonnaise slathered over it, and eating tons of it herself, as much for the emotional comfort as the meager nutritional value.

A few years later, Elizabeth weighed enough to be the brunt of cruel teasing. "I didn't do much except eat and cry myself to sleep," she told me. "I was so lonely, and my mother was never there."

In high school, Elizabeth started to run with a crowd of "misfits," as she called them, who bolstered each other's egos by sneering at the popular kids and drinking large quantities of beer. Elizabeth didn't think of them as friends but as buffers against an even crueler world.

By the time she moved to New York, she'd just about given up the idea of ever having any close relationships. Over the ensuing years, she became increasingly reclusive, traveling only between work and home and using food and beer for solace. She saw few people besides the one sister who lived nearby and the physician who was treating her for debilitating rheumatoid arthritis.

"I live like a mole," Elizabeth said, avoiding my gaze. "I hate people to look at me, and I hate to look at myself." Elizabeth admitted that she had thought about suicide many times. I was, she told me, the last possible hope. I realized that for Elizabeth, phentermine and fenfluramine could be lifesaving drugs, just as surely as epinephrine could be for the victim of cardiac arrest.

Elizabeth responded well to the medications, demonstrating almost no side effects and losing 8 pounds in two weeks. After just two months and the loss of 22 pounds, Elizabeth found it easier to move around and more pleasurable to look at herself in the mirror. She felt a rush of unusual feelings, such as an optimism and excitement, which had been buried by the wall of weight around her. Elizabeth bought herself new clothes in a fashionable department store and felt no guilt about the cost. "I deserve to wear something nice," she told me. "I've waited long enough."

I savored her expression of pleasure as she described her new outfits for me, and I enjoyed watching her change other aspects of her appearance, such as hairstyle and makeup. I had a feeling, though, that she was after more than superficial changes, and I was right.

Elizabeth's major transformation began about six months or so after she started the medications, when she asked a colleague to join her for lunch. Such a simple invitation might not sound like much to most of us, but to Elizabeth, it was an act of courage. Not since high school had she reached out to connect socially with a human being other than her sister. Even keeping up the rudiments of conversation—"What does your husband do?" "Have you seen any good movies lately?" —had to be practiced.

It was tough going, but a year later, Elizabeth's weight loss of 78 pounds had given her the confidence she needed to break through her isolation. After the lunch dates, she went on to enroll in an adult education course and to sign up as a volunteer with a neighborhood political club. She began to make plans for a dinner party in her small apartment. The thought of actually establishing friendships brought her close to tears.

"When the weight started to come off," she told me, "I realized how lonely I had been. It was like there was nothing standing between me and other people anymore. I saw that I could fill up the emptiness with something besides food and beer.''

As long as she remains on phentermine and fenfluramine, Elizabeth knows that there is little danger in backsliding. The predictability of the drugs provides a base that enables her to go forward and create dramatic changes in her life. Within the past year or so, Elizabeth has begun dating a divorced man she met in one of her courses. Although she describes the relationship as ''casual,'' it is clearly a major milestone for a woman who, until a few years ago, had been totally alone. No matter what direction this particular relationship takes, Elizabeth realizes she can continue to go forward in opening up her life.

The Confidence to Excel

''In my line of work, appearance counts,'' Charlie Constantino told me the first time I saw him. Charlie was in the fashion industry, a sales representative for an upscale men's-wear manufacturer. The company's advertisements featured physically fit young men, wearing its latest creations, being eyed appreciatively by attractive young women. The salesmen didn't have to be as fit as the male models, but they did have to look good. ''A dumpy salesman is a real turnoff for most retailers,'' Charlie commented sadly, ''even if the bosses don't look so great themselves.''

At age thirty-eight, Charlie was about 20 percent above his expected weight and—as far as he could remember—he'd always been that way. ''I've been dragging around these extra pounds longer than Marley's ghost dragged that chain," he complained.

It seemed to Charlie that no matter how often he fought to free himself, the pounds always won. His latest effort involved switching to a vegetarian diet and taking an aerobics class. Yet, in several months he achieved no weight loss, only a dramatic upswing in appetite that tortured him constantly.

"I'm so hungry I can't think about anything else but hamburgers," Charlie lamented. "If you don't help me, Doctor, I'm going to run straight over to McDonald's and slobber down every bit of fat in sight."

Charlie came to see me because a friend who was my patient told him I was using some medications that would control his appetite. He was at a point where he either had to lose the weight or get out of the fashion business. "There are just too many younger guys breathing down my neck," he said. It made him feel sad, though, to feel that his weight problem had robbed him of so much potential.

Charlie's first few weeks on phentermine and fenfluramine were marked by mild nausea. When I advised him to eat saltine crackers to settle his stomach, he replied that the nausea didn't bother him because the weight was coming off so fast. "Ten pounds in two weeks, that's worth a little seasickness," he joked. His only concern was that his decrease in appetite wouldn't last. I assured Charlie that he had nothing to worry about if he continued to use the medications and stuck to the rest of the program.

As the nausea lifted, and Charlie became adjusted to the medications, he experienced an unusual surge of energy and well-being, as if "someone were clearing cobwebs out of my head." The first thing he noticed was that he was looking forward to certain business trips, rather than feeling annoyed at having to undertake them. It was five years, at least, he told me, since he'd welcomed the idea of being on the road. But now, instead of focusing on the hassles, such as crowded airports and noisy hotels, he found himself warming to the challenge of making the sale, "as if I were just starting out."

Charlie felt somehow as if he had dropped years as well as pounds, and he realized how much the excess weight had aged him mentally. As his sales figures mounted, his superiors began to look at Charlie differently and to treat him with increased respect. "Looking good, Constantino," his boss said one day, and Charlie understood that the comment could be taken in more than one way.

With his weight coming under control, Charlie stopped worrying so much about those "younger guys" who were right behind him and, in his mind at least, all so much thinner. For the first time in his working life, he started to evaluate seriously where he really wanted to go. Since he lacked certain educational qualifications, he had never thought beyond staying in sales. Now he began to consider taking courses in management and marketing. Was he dreaming, he asked me, or simply waking up at last?

One of the wonders of weight loss, I told Charlie, is that it releases the capacity to catch up on old dreams. With the drugs, Charlie could feel secure about continuing to lose weight, and that was why he was ready to get on with aspects of his life he had neglected.

Charlie has since enrolled in one of the courses he was thinking about and his latest job evaluation noted that he possesses "management potential," a point that was never made about him before. Behind the evaluation is an altered

Charlie, one who thinks about himself in an expanded way. Whether or not his career advances, Charlie's psyche has taken a big step forward. He is confident enough to try for the most he can achieve in his working life.

The Confidence to Fall in Love

"My weight doesn't hold me back at all," Sybil Thomas told me with a smile, while detailing her active life and trying to find out if we had any acquaintances in common besides the colleague who had referred her to me. Sybil, a successful banker, was widely known for her cheery nature, which was apparent to me even as we chatted in my office. For Sybil, according to my colleague, there was no such thing as "a bad hair day." A natural networker, she enjoyed bringing people together at the social events she initiated, and she was a true friend to everyone in her wide circle.

Although Sybil was pretty modest, she admitted to always having been popular. Her weight problem had never interfered with her ability to attract people, she said, including a collection of men she described as "interesting."

Though content with her weight, Sybil, at age forty-two, had reached the point where it was interfering with her health. Ever practical, she had surveyed her network and come to me as a physician who seemed to have answers. She had heard about the miraculous results achieved by phentermine and fenfluramine. One of her current escorts, Henry Watson, was somewhat dubious about medications, but he was prepared to help her over whatever "rough spots" there might be at the beginning.

It turned out that Henry's efforts were not needed. Besides a slight drowsiness, Sybil experienced no side effects, and the weight started to come off rapidly. What surprised me was that some of Sybil's cheeriness disappeared along with the weight. Rather than being pleased by the loss, she was apprehensive. "It doesn't quite feel like me," she said with a nervous laugh.

Sometimes when a person has been overweight for a long time, it's difficult to look in the mirror and recognize the thinner image of oneself. Still, most people adapt quickly enough and are usually delighted. What exactly was making Sybil so uncomfortable?

One of the things she told me was that she was seeing a lot more of Henry Watson than she had in the past. I wondered if his response to the change in her was sabotaging her efforts in some way. What I didn't realize was that Sybil was undergoing a transformation experience—and she was fighting it.

All her life, she'd been using her personality to attract people to her and her excess weight to keep men from getting too close. The greater the number of "escorts" on her list, the less she risked falling in love with any one of them. On a certain level, Sybil understood all this and cultivated it. On another level, she yearned for love, which she equated with something that could only happen to a thinner self.

Her weight loss thrilled her more than she was willing to admit, yet terrified her. She saw that the barrier she had depended on to protect her feelings was being eroded. But as Sybil continued to use the medications, the balance tipped, as it usually does, in favor of the transformation process. After four months or so, she sensed a desire to stop the social merry-go-round she had created and to focus on this one special and quiet relationship.

Rather than resenting Henry Watson's heightened attentions, she allowed the loving and comforting aspects of his presence into her life. As her emotional horizons expanded, so did her sense of confidence at being a person who could seek and accept love. When she looked in the mirror, she began to recognize the new, thinner person she saw as herself.

The last time I saw Sybil, she and Henry were making plans to rent a Tuscan villa together for a month's vacation. "You know," Sybil told me, "I've never been alone with someone that long before." She didn't sound the least bit apprehensive.

Transformation—and Beyond

These stories illustrate the truly transforming nature of weight loss.

Until the advent of phentermine and fenfluramine, it wasn't really possible to concentrate on the possibilities of transformation because weight loss itself was, for most people, an ephemeral thing. Weight that was gone today could come back tomorrow, destroying the emotional benefits of whatever had been achieved, and leaving the dieter more depressed than ever.

How could a person begin to think about gaining the confidence to feel comfortable with food, to make emotional connections, or to consider new career directions when he or she was still vulnerable to the hunger pangs that, almost inevitably, led to regained weight?

With the medications, weight loss has become, for the first time, a dependable process with lasting results. These drugs not only open up the possibility for permanent change, but produce new attitudes toward eating and exercise so that the full power of these weight-loss foundations can be actualized. A new excitement develops. An empowering rebirth occurs. In the next few chapters, I'll demonstrate how the drugs make alterations in eating habits and the ability to exercise not only satisfying but pleasurable.

CHAPTER SIX

Becoming a Food-Aware Eater

In a study by a Penn State nutritionist, 72 subjects—some overweight and some of normal weight—were given a cup of yogurt to eat a half-hour before lunch. All yogurts were the same volume, tasted alike, and had the same number of calories. One of the surprising results of this experiment was that the men of normal weight who said they weren't concerned about gaining weight actually consumed fewer calories during the ensuing luncheon than other test subjects, including those overweight people who said they were watching how much they ate. The men who ate sparingly, the researcher concluded, seemed to have some kind of physiological edge. The researcher defined it as an internal mechanism that rapidly detects the energy content of foods and then triggers an unconscious adjustment of the number of calories consumed: in short, an early warning system that adds up to an almost instinctive ability to make the right eating choices, without any sense of deprivation.

All overweight people have noticed the existence of this mechanism in some thin people they know. It's what patients mean when they tell me, with envy in their voices, about friends who "can eat anything they want and not gain weight." My patients fail to notice that although their friends can eat "anything," they are probably not eating very much of it, because they possess—through some kind of gift of the gods—the early warning system. This system is, of course, what my patients do not have. On the contrary, they are plagued by a crippling phenomenon that is almost the opposite: irresistible urges to eat, even when there doesn't seem to be any apparent reason to be hungry.

As I explained earlier, these urges, and the lack of satiety that accompany them, appear to be genetic in many overweight people. When I first interview patients, they almost inevitably tell me that they have "always" been hungry. They simply don't remember a time when they weren't victimized by frequent impulses to reach for food. And although they may blame themselves for being heavy, they realize on some level that nature hasn't been fair. Some people have an automatic ability not to eat too much. Others can't stop eating, no matter how hard they try. The playing field isn't level.

The wonder of fenfluramine and phentermine is that these medications even up the odds. They empower you to be more like those lucky ones who eat less without trying. True, the drugs can't give you an early warning system if you don't have one, but they can release you from the terrible urges that have made it impossible for you to guide your nutritional destiny.

They can end your obsession with food and replace it with conscious judgments. And they do it without making you feel deprived.

It's exciting to find that, for the first time, you can choose how much you eat and when. You can even utter those magic words, "I'm full." Now it seems natural and even pleasurable to eat more sensibly, because you've been released from a biochemical prison.

In the past, you probably resented being advised to follow the basics of nutrition because you knew you couldn't adhere to them, no matter how much you wanted to. When you take fenfluramine and phentermine, all of that changes. You become free to act in your own best interests. You feel a new enthusiasm for eating right, and you leave your aversion to nutrition—which comes from too much failed dieting—behind you.

An Altered Vision

If you're like most of my patients, you already know these facts about weight loss:

- How much you eat is just about the most significant variable affecting your weight.
- When you eat more calories than you expend, you gain weight.
- To lose weight, you need to decrease the number of calories you take in and increase the amount of energy you use up.

These three principles sound simple enough, but it's far from simple for overweight people to pay attention to them. It's not that they don't know what they have to do; they despair of being able to do it. So many don't want to hear about nutrition at all—particularly the "d" word, *diet.*

But fenfluramine and phentermine put an end to that, and not because they help you to adhere to a diet. The system I present to patients is not a diet, in any sense of the word. I do not stress portion control because I don't believe how much you eat is under a patient's control. Portions will be controlled, however, when the medications are used, because the medications won't let you overeat. I can say this safely because I know that phentermine and fenfluramine will make you feel satiated and satisfied—at peace with your meal and the meal that is to come. They act as a safety net that makes it just about impossible for you to overeat. Think about what that means: You experience something you've probably lacked all of your life —a sense of comfort being around food.

Although they may eat a great deal, most overweight people don't realize how uncomfortable food makes them feel. They're generally tortured by cravings, wondering how to sneak the next morsel of food, feeling guilty after they've eaten it. They even fear going to restaurants, which they view as a source of food traps.

One of my patients actually cried with joy the night all this ended. She'd been on the medications two weeks when a friend asked her to dinner at a famous New York restaurant. As they ate, my patient noticed an odd sensation. She could put her fork down before the moment she would have normally considered the meal's end. She wasn't thinking ahead to dessert. In fact, she didn't want dessert at all. And she left some of the dinner on her plate. Most startling of all, my patient thought, "I'm enjoying myself tonight."

When you're on fenfluramine and phentermine, you don't have to *do* anything to lose weight. You're not dieting. You're free to enjoy yourself, even eating some foods you know are bad for you because of their fat or caloric content. As your body gets into better biochemical balance, it seeks out its natural nutritional interests. Let me show you how this works.

When I first met Alvin Tyler, a painting contractor, he told me that he hated nutritionists. "I've burned just about every diet book I ever bought," he told me. "They do more for the fireplace than they ever did for me." But within forty-eight hours of starting on the medications, Alvin noticed that his urge to eat indiscriminately was gone. At first it felt funny, as if a part of him had disappeared. He kept waiting for the obsessions to return. Alvin was accustomed to reaching for candy, a cookie, or a leftover from dinner when the urges came over him. But now, he could go from one meal to another without snacking, and he didn't feel the least bit deprived. Even before bedtime, which was when Alvin's food urges had always been at their strongest, he didn't want anything to eat.

As his mind cleared of obsessions, there seemed to be room for more productive thoughts. It was as if there were a space waiting to be filled up with common sense. "I was doing so good," Alvin told me, "I wondered if I couldn't do even better if I helped things along." Alvin rescued the one book he hadn't destroyed and looked through it. He noticed a sentence he had underlined many times. It said that to lose weight you have to take in fewer calories than you use up in energy. Now, Alvin was ready to listen.

Facing Some Facts

When patients like Alvin arrive at the listening point, I feel a sense of excitement because I know the attitudinal shift is going to help them succeed. A practical attitude is important in weight loss since overweight people are not generally very realistic about how to help themselves or even how much they eat. This was graphically demonstrated a few years ago in an experiment at St. Luke's–Roosevelt Hospital Center in New York City. Researchers tracked the eating patterns of 10 significantly overweight people, all of whom claimed to eat less than 1,200 calories a day and blamed their weight on faulty metabolism. The doctors found that the subjects were actually eating more than 2,000 calories a day—nearly twice as much as they believed—and all had normal metabolisms.

This experiment demonstrates how food obsessions can distort your judgment and perception of caloric intake. But in a land filled with high food consumption, it's easy to fall into the "I really don't eat so much" trap. The average American consumes 2,175 pounds of food a year, and eats a diet of 3,600 calories a day, compared with a worldwide average of 2,700. Everywhere you look, people seem to be snacking on pizza, hot dogs, or ice cream. Since everyone else is doing it, you join in, and you lose track of how much you are eating. Nutritional planning begins with getting a handle on what is really happening.

One way to start is to keep a food diary for a week or two, writing down everything you eat and drink, both at mealtimes and in between. It's a good idea to keep a small notebook and pencil with you so that the diary will be complete. One objective is to see how much you eat. Another is to find out which types of foods you favor. Put a star next to those foods that contain a high proportion of sugar (such as cookies) or fat (such as bacon and bologna) or alcohol. These are foods you will want to work on curtailing, particularly if you eat or drink large amounts of them.

Also note where you do your eating. Some types of restaurants—those that feature buffets, for example—can encourage higher food intake. So can certain rooms in your house. The kitchen, particularly for the cook, is an obvious hazard, but for many people so is the room where television viewing takes place. Other people find their offices, either at home or at work, to be trouble spots.

It's also important to determine which foods seem to trigger increased eating. You may notice, for example, that your list grows longer after eating certain breads, a piece of cheese, or candy. Although triggers usually have a high fat or sugar content, they can vary from one person to another. Alvin Tyler, for example, discovered that he always ate more after munching on carrots. A few of my patients have found that carbohydrates trigger their appetites. For these individuals, I often suggest restriction of carbohydrates such as pastas, breads, and other starches, or to limit these food items to one meal per day.

What's crucial is to know your particular patterns. Once they have been determined, you can work toward changing your nutritional approach.

Definitely Not Dieting

We know that regimented diets do not work. In fact, obesity experts have concluded that 95 percent of all diets are useless because they are too restrictive. Although people may lose weight, the rigidity encourages them to revert to their old patterns after the weight is gone. In short, a diet can be just about as oppressive as food obsessions.

I don't talk about diet with patients. Instead, I put forth a number of nutritional options, beginning with the idea of the limited variety system. This system can be used either to jump start a nutritional program or as a permanent approach. Limited variety is based on the startling discovery that you can eat as much as you want and still lose weight, as long as you limit your selections to three or four foods per meal. These can even be the same foods at every meal if that is your preference.

The Magic of Limited Variety

Did you ever notice how much more you eat when you're standing in front of a buffet table? Even if you're determined not to eat too much, the bountiful display triggers what I call "curiosity eating." You just want to see what a certain food tastes like. Or, you wonder if it's prepared just the way Mama used to make it. Or, you may not have had the dish for a long time, and you ask yourself if it's still made the same way. No wonder one of my patients described weddings, bar mitzvahs, and other celebrations as "a war zone where you just can't win."

Quite often, people blame themselves for having "pigged out" at a food-laden party. But there's a physiological reason for what happens. Too many choices lead to confusion about real hunger and make it difficult to control appetite. Apparently, when lots of foods are provided, the normal biochemical intervals between eating and feeling full become lengthened. In short, it takes the brain longer to tell you that you have had enough to eat. Typically, you may not feel full until twenty minutes after you've eaten the last of your buffet choices. By this time, you are more than full—you are stuffed.

Even a small amount of variety can increase appetite. For example, if you told me you were hungry, and I served you a number of Chinese dumplings, you would eat until you were satisfied. But if I then brought out fried rice, you would get hungry again and eat the rice as well. You might even finish off any dumplings you had left over.

In our society, food variety is all around us. It's difficult even to order a hamburger without having it served with french fries, cole slaw, and so forth. The rule you need to remember is this: The more types of food are included in a meal, the more you are going to want to eat. This is why you have to practice defensive eating by limiting variety.

I offer my patients guidelines in this area, but I make it very clear that I don't want them to feel hemmed in or obsessive in following my advice. Limited variety means eating only three or four foods per meal, but it doesn't mean limited amounts. You can eat as much of these foods as you want. I ask my patients to get up in the morning and think about the meals they want to eat that day, mentally select the foods, and resolve to stick with them. If they want to, they can eat the same foods at every meal.

A typical limited-variety menu would be fruit, cereal, milk, and coffee for breakfast; tuna fish, tomatoes, a vegetable, and bread for lunch, and chicken breast, a vegetable, a salad, and a baked apple for dinner. You may find that not combining proteins (meat, fish, poultry) and carbohydrates (potatoes, bread, rice, pasta) at dinner is a simple way of limiting variety.

With limited variety, it's just about impossible not to lose weight. Even if you choose to eat chocolate cake, pizza, and soda, for example, I am confident that the medications will allow you to resist the temptation to overeat. The drugs are, in effect, your secret weapon against overconsumption.

Another point is that with the medications, highly fattening foods simply lose their thrill. You don't crave them, so you don't feel compelled to select them. And eating in a balanced manner—the cornerstone of your food life from now on—becomes not only sensible but pleasurable.

Personalized Systems

Balanced eating is based on making appropriate selections—in short, being food aware. "But isn't 'food awareness' just another phrase for being on a diet?" a patient once asked me. Not at all. Food awareness is the very opposite of blind dieting because it comes from within. In fact, it seems to be part of that extra edge that naturally thin people have developed without trying too hard.

Some thin people seem to be able to eat anything and never gain weight. But many slim people constantly make food choices. If they've had a big meal the night before, they have a light breakfast. If they know they'll be having a big dinner, they opt for a lighter lunch. If their clothing feels a bit tight, they cut back slightly until the clothes fit comfortably again. If they find three average meals are too much for them, they eat four or five mini-meals throughout the day.

It's no trick for them and, even for you, the only trick is to realize that you have to pay more attention to develop this awareness. But although the job may be different, it isn't hard at all, particularly when fenfluramine and phentermine have curtailed your cravings and opened your mind.

I work with my patients to help them personalize eating systems because no single approach can apply to everyone. An eating style must be yours alone and must be consistent with lifestyle. For example, let's consider two of my patients whose daily routines were quite different.

Doris Lindsay was a stay-at-home mom with two small children. Her eating pattern was to snack throughout the day and eat along with the kids, routinely finishing the food they left, even though the medication had put her food cravings pretty much under control. Habit is, of course, the legacy of the cravings, and it can be just as difficult to deal with.

I told Doris that her first priority was to stop finishing the children's food. She had to toss out the leftovers, no matter how guilty this made her feel, and tell herself that the kids had eaten them. This innocent pretense was necessary for her own nutritional survival.

I advised Doris to wait until the children were playing quietly or napping before preparing her own midday meal and sitting down to eat it, no matter what time of day it happened to be. She was to take the phone off the hook and make mealtime her own time to relax and unwind. I also suggested that she and her husband keep the children company at dinner but hold off on eating their own dinner until the kids had gone to bed. This way, meals would be special and separate from the blur of all-day snacking that had been Doris's downfall. To avoid getting too hungry if meals were delayed, I told Doris to keep a supply of low-calorie snacks, such as fresh fruit, carrot and celery sticks, or baked fat-free corn chips.

Sam Kramer, a productivity consultant, had no trouble at home, but during his once-a-month business trips, he ate to the hilt in restaurants, often calling more dinner meetings than were necessary so that he could enjoy a variety of local eateries.

Like Doris's, Sam's food cravings had diminished, yet he still had difficulty maintaining healthy eating habits in restaurants. Sam needed to create an on-the-road eating environment that gave him the option of avoiding restaurants.

I suggested that Sam book hotels that had refrigerators in the rooms or, better yet, small kitchenettes. This would allow him to keep on hand a supply of staple foods, such as fresh fruits, cereals, whole-grain bread, low-fat yogurt, juices, and bottled water, if he wanted to have breakfast in his room, or even occasional lunches.

What happens on the road is that people feel they're losing out if they don't partake of the array of food choices around them. But their own lack of control makes them anxious and unhappy. By establishing his own "food oasis" in the hotel, limiting variety and limiting his fat intake, Sam could maintain his mental equilibrium and eat well at the same time.

Food systems need to be adapted as your personal situation changes. When Doris returned to work, for example, she revised her schedule so that she and her husband could have dinner with the kids.

It's also important to break out of the mold once in a while, just for fun and to see that you can survive it. I tell my patients that they can even eat fattening foods occasionally. The medication safety net is always there to prevent overindulgence.

Getting in Balance

Personalized as they may be, all good eating plans focus on a low-fat, low-calorie regimen that is balanced according to the recommendations of the Department of Agriculture. Fifteen percent of calories should come from protein, 25 to 30 percent from fat, and 60 percent from carbohydrates, particularly complex carbohydrates.

Think of foods rich in complex carbohydrates—carbohydrates without any sugar added—as the high-test fuel needed to perform daily activities. This is why more than half your diet should derive from these sources, which include breads, rice, pasta, potatoes, fruits, and vegetables. When eaten in their natural state, carbohydrates are not only low in fat and high in fiber, they are loaded with nutrients. It's a good idea to center each of your meals around these so-called plant foods. Try to purchase them as close to consumption as possible to ensure freshness and maximal nutritional value.

All carbohydrates are transformed by the body into glucose, a form of sugar carried through the blood by insulin and transported to the cells for energy. Glucose not used by the cells is stored in the muscles and the liver in the form of glycogen. But since less than a pound can be stored this way, remaining glucose is converted to body fat. There's no need to be alarmed by this fact. Ounce for ounce, carbohydrates are no more fattening than proteins. Still, a great deal of inaccurate information has been published in the press recently.

One New York newspaper announced in a sensational front-page story that eating pasta and other starches is a major cause of weight gain in the United States. The report said that a small group of insulin-resistant people respond to carbohydrates by overproducing glucose, thus increasing stores of fat. The implication was that carbohydrates will make you fat, even if you are not insulin resistant. Reputable nutritionists quickly pointed out that there were no significant studies to support this claim. Still, my phone rang off the hook as anxious patients called for advice.

My response was that there was no reason to stop relying heavily on carbohydrates. In addition to the other good things they do, carbs have a high water content and relatively few calories. They give you energy, and the most reliable evidence shows that they do not make you fat—unless, of course, you consume an excessive amount.

It should be noted that I do have a few patients who seem to become hungrier after eating carbohydrates, especially simple or refined carbohydrates. It is these individuals who need to limit how much carbohydrates they eat and may be better served by changing the timing of meals with carbohydrates until later in the day.

The reputation of carbohydrates as an appropriate nutritional cornerstone remains undiminished. While you're eating your carbs, don't ignore that 15 percent of calories from protein. The best way to meet this requirement is to eat small amounts of fish, poultry, or lean red meat every day.

Fat Busting

About 37 percent of the total calories in the average American diet come from fat. And gram for gram, dietary fat contains more than twice the calories of protein and carbohydrates.

One of the most effective ways to reduce caloric intake, without making any other dietary changes, is to eat less fat. But that's not always easy to do. About half of dietary fat comes from "invisible" sources, such as the animal fats and vegetable oils used in various products, especially packaged goods.

When it comes to fats, your food awareness needs to be turned up high. A good way to raise awareness is to read the labels of packaged and canned foods before you purchase them. Thanks to the Food and Drug Administration, commercially packaged foods now come with labels that are designed to provide you with accurate information about the food. The *Nutrition Facts* label now includes a column called "% Daily Value" or "% DV." This lets you know at a glance what percentage of the day's daily allotment of calories and fat a food contains.

Check the label on page 108. This sponge cake has 1 gram of fat, or 2 percent of the daily value, which is safely below your recommended 30-percent goal. Now, look at the bottom of the label and you'll see the guide for how much of each key nutrient you should have each day based on either a 2,000- or 2,500-calorie diet.

You may still find it hard to resist fatty foods, since they're full of substance, aroma, and taste. So you have to develop a strategy for cutting back. It can help to remember that you don't have to eliminate fat entirely, just keep it under 30 percent of your food plan.

You can skim fat from your meals by choosing fruits and vegetables; dried beans, peas, and lentils; grain foods like bread, bagels, and English muffins; rice, pasta, and most breakfast cereals; and sensible portions of fat-trimmed fish, chicken, turkey, and lean meats.

Nutrition Facts

Serving Size: ¼ sponge cake (50 g)
Servings per Container: 4

AMOUNT PER SERVING

Calories	160	Calories from fat 10

		% Daily Value*
Total Fat	1 g	2%
Saturated Fat	0 g	0%
Cholesterol	30 mg	10%
Sodium	70 mg	3%
Total Carbohydrate	33 g	11%
Dietary Fiber	1 g	4%
Sugars	19 g	
Protein	3 g	

Vitamin A	2%	Vitamin C	0%
Calcium	2%	Iron	4%

* Percent Daily Values are based on a 2,000-calorie diet. Your daily values may be higher or lower depending on your calorie needs.

	Calories	2,000	2,500
Total Fat	Less than	65 g	80 g
Saturated Fat	Less than	20 g	25 g
Cholesterol	Less than	300 mg	300 mg
Sodium	Less than	2,400 mg	2,400 mg
Total Carbohydrate		300 g	375 g
Fiber		25 g	30 g

Calories per Gram:
Fat 9   Carbohydrates 4   Protein 4

Try eating "low-fat" versions of staples, such as reduced-fat mayonnaise, yogurt, ice cream, milk, and cheese. Some people find these products totally satisfying. Others discover that they merely trigger a desire for the full-fat original. If that happens to you, it's best to go "cold turkey" on certain foods. As long as you get enough calcium from other sources, for example, you don't really need to have cheese in your eating plan.

Another thing to remember is that low-fat ice creams and cookies can be quite high in calories if they contain plenty of sugar. Low-fat doesn't necessarily mean low cholesterol either, since cholesterol and fat aren't the same thing. So be wary and read the labels before you buy.

One thing you needn't do, though, is to count calories. Focus your food plan on reducing fat and selecting complex carbohydrates and you take care of the calorie problem automatically. Once you eat this way, and maintain your medication schedule, it would be a real trick for you to fail to lose weight.

Alternate Eating Systems

The high-fat content of the Western diet is unusual. In most non-Western countries, only 10 to 25 percent of calories comes from fat, generally in the form of unsaturated vegetable fats. People eat a semivegetarian diet, depending heavily on the carbohydrates found in grains and with most protein coming from plant foods.

Adopting a diet of this type is an excellent way to cut down on saturated fat and cholesterol and to improve overall health. Studies have shown that the incidence of cancer, heart disease, and other chronic ailments is lower in countries where the diet includes only small amounts of animal products, such as meats and dairy foods. The obesity rate can be so low as to be insignificant.

In rural China, for example, most people are trim because 70 percent of their diet comes from carbohydrates, primarily rice. The Japanese diet is also carbohydrate based, with protein calories derived from fish and soy products.

If they are interested, I urge my patients to join the majority of the world when it comes to nutrition. My only caution is not to go too low in fat consumption. A figure like 10 percent is unrealistic for most Americans, and it can be dangerous, too. The side effects of super-low-fat diets—unless they're done under a doctor's supervision—can include menstrual dysfunction, iron deficiencies, growth retardation, and bone disorders.

Many patients ask about the advisability of following a vegetarian diet. I point out that such a plan is no guarantee of losing weight. Over the years, I've treated many 300-pound vegetarians. While many vegetarians eat low-fat, low-cholesterol foods, others eat plenty of eggs, fatty cheeses, whole milk, nuts, and seeds. They also tend to eat cookies, potato chips, pretzels, and other high-fat snacks, thus consuming as many calories as nonvegetarians.

When I first met Hillary Jackson, she was just such a high-fat vegetarian. "I believe in vegetarianism on principle," she told me, "but I find that the vegetables taste better when I put butter and cheese on them. That's the taste I really seem to crave."

Hillary, who weighed 284 pounds, was determined to lose weight, but she was deeply troubled by food urges that seemed to be beyond her control. Phentermine and fenfluramine subdued these cravings, and Hillary worked on taking the fat out of her vegetarian diet.

To begin making changes, Hillary started using low-calorie, fat-free margarine on her vegetables. Then she expanded her diet to include more whole-grain breads and cereals, legumes (such as soybeans, sprouts, chickpeas, and lentils), nuts, seeds, and fortified soybean products. With my encouragement, Hillary went to the library and discovered a greater number of vegetarian cookbooks than she had imagined. The intriguing recipes made it easier to add interest to her daily fare. If you want to adopt a vegetarian or semivegetarian eating plan, look over such books. Decide if the recipes appeal to you. If they don't, you're not likely to be very happy.

If you decide to go ahead, proceed slowly. Begin by substituting cereal, vegetables, or fruit for meat once or twice a week. Then increase the substitutions until you are no longer eating meat. If you don't want to eliminate all flesh, exchange animal meats for fowl or fish. Lacto-ovo-vegetarians—those who eat no meat or fish but do eat dairy products and eggs—have an easier time getting a full range of nutrients.

VLCD

When a patient is severely obese—140 percent over suggested body weight—and has a health risk, I usually suggest a very-low-calorie diet (VLCD) of 500 to 800 calories before starting on the medications. Such a program must be physician supervised and of short duration, usually one to two weeks. The purpose is to reduce health risks and jump-start long-term weight loss.

I usually prescribe a protein formula—such as Optifast or

H.M.R.—three to five times a day. These liquid meals contain up to 50 grams of carbohydrate, up to 100 grams of protein, vitamins, minerals, and trace elements, and very small amounts of fats. To ensure adequate protein, I recommend that the patient also eat small portions of white meat turkey, tuna, cod, or shrimp.

With these rapid weight-loss programs, there are potential dangers. Patients may feel light-headed or dizzy and blood pressure may drop. Another potential danger is the development of gallstones.

If your physician puts you on a VLCD, you'll be told to drink 2 liters of water a day in order to prevent dehydration and other complications. You'll also be asked to notify the doctor should you experience any troublesome physical symptoms.

Any physician will also tell you what I'm going to say now: Do not put yourself on such a diet. Although there are commercial products you can buy, the health risks without medical supervision are severe, particularly for teenage girls, who are the most likely to try this type of diet. Possible side effects include growth retardation, loss of lean body mass, cardiac changes, and electrolyte imbalances.

If you are on a VLCD, remember that it is just a transitional eating program. For health reasons, you need to lose weight rapidly. But even as you sip your lunch, try to avoid becoming overly dependent on a method of weight loss that makes decisions for you. In the real world of the supermarket and the refrigerator, you'll need to make your own food choices. If you follow the guidelines in this chapter, you should have no difficulty.

Do You Need a Nutritionist?

Some patients relish the challenge of constructing their own eating plans. There are countless books available that provide detailed information on low-fat foods and low-fat cooking, for example. Others are just as interested in making changes, but feel they lack a sense of direction—they want expert guidance hand-tailored to their specific needs. These are the people who can benefit from the services of a nutritionist—a professional who provides personalized diet planning, instruction, and modification.

Your first session with a nutritionist may start with a physical assessment, including height, weight, height/weight ratio, and body fat composition. Blood tests may also be recommended to check for nutritional deficiencies.

At my recommendation, Doris Lindsay, the homemaker I told you about earlier, consulted with Susan Taman Levy, a registered dietitian who is part of my treatment team and is also affiliated with New York University Medical Center. When Susan asked Doris to define what she thought good nutrition was, she got vague statements like "eating less." Susan also learned that Doris believed in quite a few nutrition myths, such as "low-fat foods have no calories in them." So Susan reviewed the major points of nutrition with Doris and also gave her handouts and pamphlets to read. Since Doris didn't know how much food she ate every day, Susan suggested keeping a food diary.

Susan also talked with Doris about her level of physical activity, so that she could gauge the calories Doris needed to lose weight and still be healthy. It took only a few sessions for

Susan, working with Doris's preferences, to design a nutrient-dense, balanced food plan that was easy to follow.

Many of my patients are amazed at how quickly nutritionists can get them started and how much motivation they can provide. Finding one may not be easy, though, since half the states have no licensing procedures or standards. This has led to a booming business for unqualified nutritional "experts."

I'd advise restricting your search to registered dietitians (RDs). An RD has a four-year degree in nutrition and has passed the registration examination given by the American Dietetic Association. Your physician or a teaching hospital may be able to suggest names in your area, or contact the referral network of the American Dietetic Association (216 West Jackson Boulevard, Chicago, IL 60606-6995; tel. 800-366-1655). Expect to pay at least $50 an hour for individual counseling, less for group counseling, if it's available.

Whether you consult a nutritionist, or work on your own to develop an eating plan, you are going to find that you have entered a new and far more rewarding stage in your relationship with food. You will also realize that this stage is going to be permanent. Your days as a failed dieter—indeed, as a dieter of any sort—are over, if you have the courage to shift your thinking out of the crippling diet mode. In a later chapter, we'll see just how to make that happen.

CHAPTER SEVEN

Exercise: Weight Loss as a Turning Point

You can lose up to 15 percent of your body weight just by taking fenfluramine and phentermine. But to stop there would be to miss the point, and to fail to get the most out of these remarkable medications, which can create a total change in your health profile.

Exercise is good medicine. I'm not talking about strenuous exercise necessarily, but simply a moderate addition to what you are doing now. If you follow the lead of the drugs, and start to move around more, you will discover advantages beyond weight loss, such as changes in the way you relate to your own body. The drugs set off a mechanism that makes it easier, and even inviting, to put more exercise in your life.

They help counter the resistance that many overweight people feel toward exercise by allowing them to appreciate the sheer pleasure of movement. They also allow the individual to concentrate more fully on what he or she is doing. This sense of complete involvement is almost impossible to give up.

The drugs ratchet up your exercise potential. No longer do you simply "endure" exercise, you appreciate it, and you recognize the increased sense of mastery it can provide over your life. A major advantage is that exercise tends to make the weight loss you achieve permanent. When I speak on the telephone with a patient who lost weight years ago and learn that he or she is still exercising, I know that the weight has not come back without seeing it for myself.

Another advantage is that the contemplative nature of exercise—the "time out" you experience being alone with your own body—makes it easier to solve problems, to be creative, and to change certain destructive behaviors. I've found that many people are able to successfully quit smoking when they begin to exercise.

One of my patients, a college physics professor, was a heavy smoker until he gave up taking the subway and began walking to work. At first, he found it slow going, but as he fell into the special rhythm of his daily walks, all kinds of ideas emerged that had been beneath the surface of his consciousness. Some were related to a physics problem he'd been trying to solve for months, but others, to his surprise, were about ways he could avoid reaching for a cigarette.

Although this man had wanted to quit for some time, he had never thought he could succeed. Nor had he ever felt so focused. Now, when he put some of his thoughts into practice, he found that they worked rather easily. Within months of starting his walks, the professor was no longer a smoker.

The Anti-Exercise Reflex

Despite the advantages, exercise can be a hard sell on my part. That's because people who have experienced repeated weight-loss failures tend to associate exercise with a losing situation.

One of my patients, for example, remembered trying to keep up with a water-dance class full of women who were in better shape than she was. "I couldn't even fit my arm into their bathing suits," she told me, "and, of course, I always lagged behind getting from one end of the pool to the other. I felt humiliated by the whole thing."

An experience like this one conditions people to react to exercise with alarm and dismay. Unfortunately, they are totally unaware of how wonderful exercise can make them feel once they break through the barriers. Thus, no matter how much I rave about the benefits of a nice walk on a spring day or a bike ride on an autumn morning, some patients come up with a long list of reasons not to do these things. I hear statements like:

"Please don't talk to me about exercise. I hate it."

"Exercise gives me a pain."

"I have no time to exercise."

"It's boring to exercise."

"I get enough exercise on my job."

I don't counter every single one of these explanations, but I do stress the advantages of movement, and I try to explain that lack of exercise is part of a universal social change. Unless they are working as lumberjacks or laborers, most people perform jobs today that aren't physical enough to count as exercise, which is why most Americans are in such sorry physical shape.

As we noted earlier, according to government surveys, less than 25 percent of us are as active as we should be, and more than half are just about completely sedentary. A sedentary life-style has been linked to as many as 250,000 deaths a year, or 12 percent of all deaths. The Centers for Disease Control and Prevention has declared an "epidemic of physical inactivity," which is just as detrimental to health as smoking and high cholesterol levels.

When it comes to not exercising, women are just as guilty as men. One survey found that 73 percent of women don't exercise enough, with older women—those over sixty-five—most likely to be the couch potatoes.

The challenge to all Americans, and to overweight people in particular, is to become more active—because if they do not, they cannot succeed long term in maintaining weight loss. I tell my patients that they have to create tasks for themselves that will replace the physical effort removed from their lives by modern conveniences like elevators and automobiles.

The power of exercise in weight loss has been proven over and over again. In a recent study at Baylor University, for example, a program as simple as walking for forty-five minutes five times a week proved to be the major factor in keeping weight off after successful weight loss.

Rethinking Exercise

In my weight-loss program, exercise and medications go hand in hand because they reinforce one another. The trick, I tell patients, is to let the medications work for them.

Because the drugs halt food cravings, and create a quick weight loss, they make people feel like they're getting somewhere. Some patients feel a sudden inspiration to increase the amount of movement in their lives. Others may sense that feeling, yet put a damper on it. The resistance stems from past experiences.

The first step is to tell yourself that this time everything is on your side. You are not going to be asked to do anything beyond your capacity because, as I will explain later, you will be the one to decide what you do, how much, and when. You are not going to be tested or judged, merely encouraged to succeed at something your body is aching to do. The next step is to take a hard look at the most common reason given for not exercising: "I haven't any time."

People's lives today are very complicated. They have to commute to and from work, fix dinner, and attend to family matters—more than enough to think about. But if the President of the United States can find time to run three or four times a week, anyone can make time for some type of exercise. I don't know how the President accomplishes this, but for most people it's a matter of establishing priorities and making hard choices that put their health first. For some patients this is very difficult to do, because they think that putting themselves first is "selfish." What they need to realize is that selfishness can actually be in the best interests of the people they love.

Roger Albertson had lost 30 pounds on the medication and made some headway toward correcting an incipient heart problem when he told me he had "no time to exercise." He had decided to take the drugs, he said, because he was too busy to bother with either exercise or nutrition. A forty-two-year-old stock analyst, he detailed a full day that began with an hour's commute and a 7 A.M. arrival at his office. "If I have to get up any earlier to exercise," he said, "I might as well not go to bed at all."

Roger got home around 7:30 P.M., ate a hurried dinner, and tried to devote the evening to helping his oldest son with his homework while his wife attended to the toddler. "I hardly spend any time with the kids," he told me, "and my son has been having a hard time with math."

For Roger, helping with homework was a sacred task, and he resisted my suggestion that he use some of this time to exercise. But when we reviewed his medical records, one point became clear: If Roger didn't start to become more "selfish," his son might not have him around for very long. When Roger realized what the choices were, he arranged for a tutor to work with his son after school, so that he could be free to exercise in the evening.

My point is that you have to first consciously block out time for yourself, no matter how much effort it takes. Making this choice signals your commitment to yourself—and your loved ones—that your health can no longer be overlooked.

"How Much Exercise Do I Need?"

My patients often ask how much exercise they need to do every day to lose weight and to keep it from coming back on. I explain that it's confining to think of exercise in such absolute terms because exercise is a highly personal matter. Still, I can't help having an ideal in mind, and that is to exercise aerobically —walking, running, swimming, or bicycling—for an hour or so three times a week and to perform at least one session of resistance training a week.

Resistance training, also called weight lifting, develops muscles that have been diminished by weight loss. Most people are surprised to learn that after they diet a while, the body burns muscle instead of fat to conserve fat stores. That is why depleted muscles need to be strengthened.

Several years ago, a panel of experts released new guidelines based on the goal of improving health rather than achieving maximum fitness. Thus was born "Exercise Lite," which, I believe, is a sensible beginning for most of my patients, particularly those who have developed resistance to exercise.

In an Exercise Lite program, you simply include a total of thirty minutes of moderate activity in your day. Even such activities as gardening, house cleaning, or walking up a flight or two of stairs can lower your risk for coronary artery disease and other chronic illnesses. So can ordinary walking, which is one of nature's great fat burners.

If you've been inactive, the advantage of Exercise Lite is that it allows you to get moving again without feeling daunted. No superhuman effort of dedication, money, or equipment is required. And, you don't have do any given activity for a full thirty minutes. Short periods of varied activities, interspersed throughout the day, provide the same health benefits. The important thing is to keep track in some way so that you neither exhaust yourself nor do too little.

Emma Cooper was one of those over-sixty-five women who fit into the "couch potato" category. Although she had entered retirement with enthusiasm, two years into it she found herself cutting back on activities she had previously enjoyed simply because she lacked structure in her day. It seemed easier to sit and stare at the television set than to plan what to do. But when Emma started losing weight on the medications, she felt an urge to get moving again, which I encouraged by explaining Exercise Lite.

Emma started by increasing the number of cleaning tasks she performed. For example, she decided to vacuum the living room carpet every day instead of twice a week, whether the carpet needed it or not. She increased the number of shopping trips she made, carrying smaller amounts of purchases, and using the steps instead of the elevator. And because she wanted to do "fun" things, too, she undertook some regular baby-sitting assignments for a working mother who lived in her building. Playing with an active toddler definitely added to Emma's exercise level.

These are just a few of the ways health-giving activities can be incorporated into a daily routine. Other activities could include raking the yard and gardening, using the stairs rather than the elevator at work, walking at least part of the way to work, riding a bike to the store instead of using the car, and carrying the laundry up the stairs from the basement. A total of fifteen minutes a day spent walking up stairs can result in a 10- to 20-pound weight loss over a year. Walking up moderate inclines, such as a hilly section of your town, can yield similar results.

As you probably noticed, the key element is to move your body and to do it consistently. Of course, there's no need to stop after thirty minutes, and when you're on the medication, you may not want to. Let your body be your guide. The more you do, the more your fitness level will zoom and your waistline will shrink.

I make it clear to my patients who have not exercised or who have not exercised with any regularity that they need to take some preliminary steps before putting on their workout clothes. Depending on your condition, your physician may recommend a complete physical as well as an exercise stress test, an important diagnostic test that is designed to uncover any cardiac abnormalities. Once you have been given a clean bill of health, your physician can design an appropriate exercise program for you, or refer you to a certified trainer.

For a patient at the lowest level of fitness, I recommend slow walking, which can burn as many as 80 calories per mile. For those interested in investing in equipment, I also recommend a cross-country ski machine like NordicTrack, an excellent exercise device that puts virtually no stress on your joints as you slide back and forth to fitness. (For the budget-conscious, there are similar machines costing as little as $150.) As you start losing weight and become stronger, the exercise intensity level can be raised and other activities introduced.

You may be perfectly happy doing nothing but Exercise Lite, and if that's the case, fine. But most patients find, as time goes on, that they want to do more. The growing sense of excitement about movement—fostered in part by the weight loss triggered by the medications—encourages this ambition. But it's important not to rush into a more structured exercise program. Instead, you need to make a number of decisions.

Finding the Right Exercise

Physicians and exercise physiologists promote programs guaranteed to produce fitness, yet only one in nine Americans exercises with any regularity. One roadblock, I believe, is that people often make the wrong exercise choices. It's not enough for me to explain all of the ways exercise will change a patient's life for the better. Unless there is a good match between the individual and the activity, exercise won't become a habit.

What can turn a potential exerciser into an actual exerciser is the selection of a program tailored to one's specific personality and interests. The exercise you embrace should in no way remind you of physical education classes if you hated them in high school. Success is much more likely to occur when you choose an activity that interested you intensely as a child, such as dancing, bike riding, swimming, or hiking. It's important to select an exercise, sport, or activity because you enjoy it, not because everyone else is doing it.

In my view, your choice should be something you can do comfortably while thinking about other things. This is what will allow you to bask in the glow of an "exercise high" and to solve personal problems, in ways similar to the college professor I told you about earlier.

What the selection of exercise really boils down to is the old adage: "Know thyself." Each of us has an individual "exercise personality." Following are five brief summaries of such personalities. Before you begin exercising, and even if you've never done any of the activities described, it's a good idea to ask yourself, "Where do I fit in?"

The Social Exerciser: You enjoy the friendly, cooperative spirit found in organized exercise classes and sporting activities. You want to have fun, and you don't care about keeping score or watching the clock. For you, the thrill comes from the camaraderie that develops from working in a group.

Suggested activities: Aerobics classes, water aerobics classes, step classes, ballroom dance classes, weight training in a gym, bicycle touring, and group walks.

The Competitive Exerciser: You're not likely to do any activity unless you have an opponent with whom you can go one-on-one. No matter what the sport, you get pumped up to play, and you play hard from start to finish. You'd rather take up a sport to get in shape than first get in shape to take up a sport, and this makes adherence to training workouts infrequent, at best. A possible downside of your competitive spirit is the increased likelihood of injury.

Suggested activities: Racquetball, tennis, volleyball, softball, basketball, bicycle racing, road racing, and competitive swimming.

The Solo Exerciser: You want to escape from people, job pressures, and daily activities—if only for an hour or so, several times a week. You value the private time to think, ponder, and plan. You also want that special dynamic of being in tune with your own body and just feeling good.

Suggested activities: Outdoors: Walking, jogging, jumping rope, bicycle riding, shooting baskets, noncompetitive swimming, and in-line skating. Indoors: Rowing machine, stairstepper, ski machine, stationary bike, and treadmill.

The Cross-trainer: You love to mix all types of exercises and sports, and you are willing to try just about anything you haven't done before. For you, experimentation is more important than expertise. What you enjoy most is facing new challenges and making new friends, particularly those who can help you expand your horizons.

Suggested activities: Weight training, cross-country skiing, triathlon competition, in-line skating, bicycle riding, swimming, and dancing.

The Nonexerciser: You avoid exercise, probably because it makes you feel self-conscious. Although you think you "hate" exercise, there may be an exerciser inside you waiting to get out. Despite your protestations, you're probably ready to try some exercise right now if you really think you might succeed.

Suggested activities: Walking, swimming, and treadmill. Last resort: Buy a dog, preferably a large one. This way you'll be sure to do some walking at least twice a day.

The Value of a Fitness Evaluation

Always consult with your physician before you start exercising. Medical clearance is recommended if you are forty or older and have not been exercising, and at any age if you have any underlying medical problems. If you have heart disease, hypertension, diabetes, or some other disease, your doctor may be able to tailor a program to your condition. If you have no obvious problem, he or she may still suggest an exercise stress test to screen for any underlying heart disease. Your physician may also perform a fitness evaluation by means of a computerized test.

I perform a fifteen-minute computerized test before my patients embark on an exercise program, and four months later I repeat the test, looking for improvements in their overall health profile. The beauty of the computerized assessment is that it lets patients see how they measure up on key components. Here are some of the things you could learn about your personal fitness level from such a test.

Body-fat composition. The percentage of body weight comprising fat is a more significant figure than bathroom scale weight. A body fat percentage of over 25 percent is too high. To lower body fat, you must reduce your intake of high-fat foods and perform regular exercise.

Muscular strength. Good muscular strength is important for physical appearance, the burning of increased calories during metabolism, prevention of back injuries, and the improvement of sports performance. You can increase your strength by doing resistance exercises two or three times a week, starting with very light weights and adding small amounts of weight every one to two weeks.

Flexibility. Good flexibility—the body's ability to move easily —is important for overall health and the prevention of injuries. Flexibility can be improved by simple stretch exercises.

Blood pressure. A continuously high blood pressure may damage arteries and lead to heart disease. Regular exercise can help to lower pressure, and if you are taking hypertension medication, exercise may allow you to reduce the medication or eliminate it all together.

Aerobic fitness. This is your level of endurance or stamina. Good aerobic fitness reduces the risk of heart disease and also helps to burn calories, assisting in both weight loss and weight maintenance. Exercises that promote aerobic fitness include brisk walking, jogging, and water running.

Keeping Tabs with Before-and-After Charts

Fitness evaluations are not only a medical tool. They also serve as an additional motivation to exercise and that is why I recommend having one done if you possibly can.

When I first reviewed Edie Meyerson's charts with her, the thirty-eight-year-old industrial engineer was quite shocked. Her body fat percentage was 37 (over 25 percent is considered high for a woman), her muscular strength was poor, she had little flexibility or stamina, and she was borderline hypertensive. I could have told Edie all of these things, but showing them to her on the computerized printout made it clear that she had to take action.

Edie then consulted with Michael Margulies, a certified personal exercise trainer, who is an indispensable part of my treatment team. Edie chose to go to Mike because she wasn't a regular exerciser and wanted one-on-one instruction that would be in a totally private setting. She also felt that the motivation she got from an exercise expert would encourage her to continue with regular workouts.

Mike showed Edie how to carry out the "get in shape"

program I had prescribed for her. This basic fitness routine I give to my patients includes daily stretching, calisthenics, light dumbbell exercises, and walking twenty minutes a day. Simple as the program was, there were dramatic improvements over the next four months.

Getting Started

I find that the best approach to fitness is consistency: Do something physical every day. You can map out your own workout routine or else work out under the watchful eye of a trainer at a local Y, health club, or fitness center.

It's always useful to have some guidelines in mind as you begin to exercise. If you are completely out of shape, short but frequent bouts of aerobic exercise, such as walking, jogging, bicycling, or aerobics classes, can dramatically improve your fitness. Be sure to build your routine gradually, but steadily, making it just a little more demanding each time you do it. Over a period of months, you will reach your optimal level of conditioning.

As you decide which forms of exercise to pursue, remember that walking, particularly for a new exerciser, is one of the safest, easiest, and least expensive things to do. About the only equipment needed is a pair of supportive, cushioned shoes. And, even though walking has a much lower level of intensity than other forms of aerobic exercise, it can still have a significant impact on health.

Walking is the most appropriate exercise for most overweight people, especially if they have high blood pressure, diabetes, or heart problems. It's easier on the joints than step classes and running, and it's just as effective. Walking three miles, for example, burns about the same number of calories as running the same distance. Running just burns the calories faster, but why be in a hurry?

I sing the praises of walking as often as I can because many people are under the mistaken impression that you have to do some gut-wrenching form of exercise to achieve benefits. That can keep them from doing anything at all.

One of my patients, Ira Lawson, came to see me because he wanted to be put on the medications. When I broached the subject of exercise, he exploded, saying that he wouldn't go anywhere near "those classes that make you jump up and down like an idiot." Even in the privacy of his own home, Ira wanted nothing to do with exercise tapes, and he had tossed out every one his wife purchased for him. "I hate exercise, that's all," he told me in a definitive tone.

I usually don't pressure people, because I know that in time phentermine and fenfluramine will begin to work their magic. That is what happened to Ira. After losing 25 pounds or so, he noticed a renewed sense of energy and vigor, accompanied by a feeling of connectedness to his own body. It was this sensation of being at home in his own skin that he wanted more of.

I explained to Ira that any exercise, even a simple exercise like walking, would give him what he yearned for—and speed up his weight loss at the same time. Ira started off slowly by taking twilight walks around his suburban block. After a few weeks, he increased his pace and lengthened his route.

As Ira became absorbed in walking and let his mind go on "automatic pilot," he noted his connectedness expanding into feelings of joy. Sometimes he found himself smiling as he walked along. It was pleasurable simply to move and to be alive. Of course, it also felt great to see the pounds coming off more quickly. Ira wanted to share his sense of excitement with his wife. She began to accompany him on his walks and they found that they were able to talk more openly than they had in years.

Ira has lost more than 100 pounds and he no longer talks about hating exercise. His experience demonstrates that exercise can be more than an instrument for losing weight. It can be a means of turning one's life around or, as in this case, a way of rediscovering some wonderful aspects of life that may have been neglected.

The Role of Resistance Training

An important form of exercise that frequently gets overlooked is resistance training, or, as it is more commonly known, weight lifting. Such training not only speeds up the loss of fat and creates a more attractive physique, it also makes you healthier. Strong muscles increase your ability to do everything, from carrying groceries to lifting your children to playing your favorite sport. Resistance training can also slow the aging process by preventing the loss of bone mass or increasing both bone mass and overall body flexibility. Paired with aerobic exercises, such as walking, running, and swimming, resistance training can further endurance and feelings of well-being.

Building muscles also helps you to lose weight because the number of calories you burn is a function of how much muscle you have. Your muscles are like an engine that is always running at some speed. As you perform resistance exercise, you burn calories. And when your muscles are at rest, even when you are sleeping, they keep burning calories. So the more muscle or lean tissue you have, the more calories you will burn at any weight, whether you are exercising or resting.

A recent study at Tufts University underscores the value of resistance training for both strength building and weight loss. Researcher Wayne Campbell put twelve sedentary men and women on a three-month weight-training program. These people did not have to lose weight, so three meals a day were provided, and those who lost a pound a day were given more food to maintain their weight.

At the end of the study, each of the subjects made dramatic strength gains, with most improving by as much as 90 percent in their legs and up to 30 percent in their arms and chest. With their metabolism boosted an extra 7 percent by the weight training, they needed an additional 300 calories a day to maintain their weight. If the subjects had been dieting and not eating the extra food, Campbell figures that each would have lost at least 10 pounds.

Resistance training is especially important for women, since they have less muscle and more fat than men. But after telling a woman that she should begin lifting weights, I can quickly tell by the look on her face that I have to counsel her. I explain that she won't get muscles like Arnold Schwarzenegger's, even after years of training. Because of hormonal differences, women can't develop bulging biceps or rippling abdominals, unless they pump iron four hours a day or take anabolic steroids. What resistance workouts will do, when performed correctly a few times a week, to give a woman a strong yet decidedly feminine look, as many delighted women have discovered.

Jenny Morris, a thirty-one-year-old retail worker, had been overweight all her life. Jenny's idea of a workout was switching channels while watching television. Her life was sedentary and totally nonathletic. But when Jenny started on fenfluramine and phentermine, she began to feel dissatisfied with her lack of movement. Like Ira Lawson, she developed a need to become reacquainted with her own body. Despite her years of practice as a couch potato, she felt increasingly restless. Somehow, with the medications, doing nothing no longer felt comfortable.

When I suggested weight lifting, Jenny laughed. She stood only five feet tall, and she thought of resistance training as something that only powerfully built men do. But she listened earnestly as I explained how the body burns muscle mass when a person diets and that weight loss at the price of weakened muscles was not our goal.

Jenny had paid a great deal of attention to her fitness evaluation, and she knew that she had little enough muscle strength as it was. Her body fat composition was at a dangerous 46 percent, a fact that had made her feel helpless, but the more we talked about weight lifting, the more excited she began to feel at the prospect of a direct attack on her problems. Resistance training, with its specific concentration on muscular buildup, might be just the physical activity she was longing for.

The day after our conversation, Jenny joined a gym near her office, and a trainer introduced her to the weight room. She showed Jenny how the various machines worked and sketched out a thirty-minute program for her to follow three days a week. As soon as Jenny started the program, she experienced a mounting sense of excitement. Although she felt clumsy at first, it soon became invigorating to perform the movements, and the process itself was fascinating to her. Jenny found that she wanted to know how muscles work, the names of the muscles, and the rationale for working one muscle group over another. She devoured the books that her trainer lent her.

"It's like going back to school," Jenny told me, "only this time, the subject is me." It had been a long time since Jenny Morris was her own major subject. A sad thing about being overweight is that it causes people to back away from their own bodies. But with the medications and the weight training, Jenny, like Ira Lawson, felt that she was reconnecting. Step by step, she saw her body transforming itself, a thrill that she found indescribable.

Jenny loved the sense of power she got from the training. Eighteen months later, she arrived at the point where she could squat with 120 pounds and bench press 95 pounds. Jenny was on top of the world. "When I leave the weight room," she said, "I feel like no one can stop me."

Jenny has lost 80 pounds and reduced her body fat composition to 19 percent. She looks terrific—trim and attractively muscular. But just as important as the powerful image Jenny projects is the strength she feels inside.

Should You Consider a Personal Trainer?

The basics of staying in shape are simple and the advice in the Resources section should get you started. Most local gyms and health clubs now have instructors who can be helpful in devising a complete exercise program. But some people will find it useful to consider a personal trainer. Because Jenny Morris was inexperienced when she started weight lifting, she benefited greatly from working with a trainer. But even long-time exercisers, like myself, can use this kind of personal attention.

I find that many patients are embarrassed to exercise in a public gym or health club by themselves because they think everyone will be looking at them. Some feel that the other members will pressure them to speed up and move along too rapidly on the equipment. These are the people who might want to consider the services of a personal trainer.

Personal trainers to the stars make headlines for keeping Hollywood's A-list looking healthy and taut. Trainers also prevent professional athletes from getting fat, and they help high-profile corporate executives achieve the body shape they need to keep their image-conscious jobs. Some trainers have even become celebrities themselves through videotape sales, endorsements, and personal appearances.

Unfortunately, the hype makes ordinary people think that trainers are only for the rich and famous. In reality, though, most personal trainers work with ordinary people who simply need help in learning how to exercise regularly and efficiently on their own. If this sounds like you, you might give some serious thought to using a trainer's services. Just as you need instruction in tennis before you go out and play, if you haven't been exercising you may need a trainer to provide techniques, coaching, helpful tips, and a good dose of motivation.

Although a trainer might seem like a luxury—fees begin at $20 an hour and can be ten times that amount in some parts of the country—if you are going to lie on the couch with a bag of chips instead of exercising, paying someone to prod you could be one of your best health investments yet. Remember that a few sessions to get started may be all you will need.

To encourage patients to think about a trainer, I sometimes

ask them to add up all the money they spend a week on food, restaurants, clothing, entertainment, and miscellaneous expenses. Somewhere there may be room to cut back so you can pay for enough sessions to move ahead comfortably with an exercise plan. It can help to think of a trainer not as a new expense, but as a lifestyle choice within your budget, if you can manage it.

When you hire a trainer, you generally exercise in the privacy of your own home, using your own equipment, or you work against the resistance supplied by the trainer. If you plan to work with a trainer on a long-term basis, you will probably have to purchase some free weights, a bench, and a step with several risers. In some instances, a client will work out with his or her trainer in the local health club, thus expanding the workout variety. If you're thinking about doing this, remember that some clubs require that you enroll as a member or that the trainer join the club. Be sure of your obligations beforehand so you won't be surprised by extra fees.

As to hiring a trainer, there are standard ways to evaluate qualifications and to find out where a trainer is available in your area. You'll find a discussion of this subject in the Resources section. In the meantime, you need to consider whether or not you want to hire an expert to train and motivate you.

Another way to motivate yourself is to seek support from a friend. The President's Council on Physical Fitness and Sports reports that such support can be critical to your success. I often recommend that my patients find someone to act as their exercise counselor. This person, preferably not a spouse, checks in regularly to see how the program is progressing. And if there are impediments, the counselor works with the exerciser to overcome setbacks.

Roger Albertson, the stock analyst I mentioned earlier who had trouble blocking out time for himself, asked a friend to phone a few nights a week to inquire about how his routine was. Just knowing that the friend would be calling inspired Roger to keep on track. Without a reminder, it's all too easy to get involved in something else or to convince yourself you'll pay more attention to exercising tomorrow.

Having a reliable workout partner is another way to ensure that you stay committed. It may be easy to come up with an excuse when only you are involved, but if it means standing up your buddy, the odds of not missing your workout improve.

In the Resources section, you will find guidelines for walking, jogging, swimming, bicycling, resistance training, and other forms of exercise. The types of exercise you prefer, and whether you do them alone, with a partner, a counselor, or a trainer, are issues you have to decide. You will know what's best if you listen to your own body and the messages the medications are giving you to get up and move.

If your inner voice isn't speaking too loudly, begin by adding Exercise Lite to your day. If you're already enthusiastic, work on developing a more serious exercise routine. If you're somewhere in between, do some Exercise Lite and some part of a routine each week.

No matter where you begin, remember that you are working your way to a better place and that exercise can be an invaluable traveling companion. Later on, when you have reached your goal, it can be the guardian of the weight loss you worked so hard to achieve. In short, start to exercise and you will become acquainted with a lifelong system of support.

CHAPTER EIGHT

Escaping the Diet Mentality

"Thinking diet every single moment is a horrible way to live," a patient once said to me. "But I don't want to be fat, so what choice do I have?" Her words made me sad because they so completely summed up the way many people have condemned themselves to live, obsessed with dieting, and without the realization that they have another choice.

Although you may well be trapped in this "horrible way to live," you don't have to be. You may believe that "thinking diet" is the only way out, but a mental preoccupation with dieting is practically guaranteed to keep you overweight. Rather than being a virtue, "diet think" actually does you a disservice.

So a primary goal is not only to get out of the diet way of acting—counting calories, exercising compulsively—but also to get out of the diet way of thinking, which I call the diet mode. The drugs can help you do this in ways I'll discuss later on in this chapter. But first, it's important to recognize what a diet mode is.

If you have any doubts that you think like a dieter, ask yourself these questions:

- Do you wake up every morning wondering how you can find the willpower to start a new diet?
- Do you scour the bookstores for the latest diet books?
- Have you tried at least five new diets in the past five years?
- Are you ashamed to tell friends you're starting yet another diet?
- Have you ever convinced yourself you were adhering to a diet when you knew you really weren't?
- Do you think you have to suffer in order to lose weight?
- Do you look forward to losing weight on a diet because then you can starting eating the way you want to again?
- Have you ever gotten through a day without envying a thin person?
- Do you hate yourself when you fail to lose weight on a diet?
- Does losing weight actually frighten you because you know it won't last?
- Does it seem like a waste of time to learn how to maintain your weight loss?

If you answered yes to any of these questions, you are caught in at least one diet mode. For as you can tell by the questions, there are several such modes, some of which may even seem harmless. But diet thinking is never harmless, even if it has become second nature to you. Let's take a close look at the modes and the dangers they pose.

Mode One

"I'm not dieting but I should be." Many overweight people spend more time ruminating about dieting than actually getting around to it. In the meantime, they wait, they worry, and they castigate themselves for lack of willpower. Doing this is like saying "I'm a bad person" to yourself every single minute. Worst of all, your relationship with food worsens because each meal is infused with a sense of impotence, making it harder to ever get started on weight loss.

Mode Two

"I'm counting on a magic formula." Some individuals collect diet tips the way others collect stock market tips. They go from one book or program to another, dabbling for a while and then deciding that something better will come along. But there is no Holy Grail of weight loss. So even though constant searching may seem productive, it can actually be a way of avoiding real action.

Mode Three

"There's something wrong with my scale." One of the worst things about dieting is that its rigidity encourages self-delusion. The more "demanding" the diet, the more you need to convince

yourself that you haven't been cheating. So you overlook the fattening foods you may have eaten or you wonder about the accuracy of your scale. Usually, if you've checked it out and you still think a scale must be faulty, the real fault lies with being in the dieting mode.

Mode Four

"I love to suffer." Often people think the best way to lose weight is to endure an excessive cutback in caloric intake. When you're in this mode, you actually relish the sense of deprivation, because you think it's working for you. But there's a reward you expect of deprivation, and that is permission to start eating heavily again after you've suffered to lose weight. This reward, by the way, is why some individuals actually get hooked on repeated dieting.

Mode Five

"I can't stop envying thin people." Although being envious seems to have little to do with dieting, it's one of the most destructive modes. Every time you believe that it's easier for a thin person to stay thin than it is for you—even if that's perfectly true— you make it more difficult to attend to your own business of losing weight. Envy is like a sign flashing "stop" to your efforts.

Mode Six

"I hate myself." Here is the most insidious mode, and it's one that grows in strength each time you fail. Self-loathing under- mines your self-esteem, makes your life a living hell, and unfor-

tunately, is almost universal among overweight people. By understanding that you may have a genetic disorder and are not at fault, you can work to put this mode behind you.

Mode Seven

"The thin me can't last." For the chronically overweight, diet thinking doesn't end when weight comes off. Instead, patients can be haunted by the idea that they will regain the weight they lost, as if they were powerless to resist. Repeated cycles of dieting reinforce a fear that's often realistic, but until you believe that you have the power to win in the end, you can't banish the specter of doubt.

Why Breaking Free Can Be Difficult

Notice that diet modes can occur before you diet, while you're dieting, and even after you have lost weight. This is one reason they are so tenacious. But what really empowers the modes is that, until now, dieting was the only weapon available to those who wanted to lose weight. A diet mentality and weight loss were synonymous, and people thought they had to "think diet" in order to succeed.

Today, with the advent of a more effective weapon—the medications—we understand how crippling the diet modes really are. And the good news is that we don't need them, because the drugs, along with the sensible eating and moderate exercise they facilitate, can do the job for us.

Still, breaking free is one of the most difficult things my patients experience because a single individual can be victimized by so many modes. Let's take Phyllis Maxwell, for example, a patient who told me that "thinking diet every single moment is a horrible way to live." Phyllis went for long periods when she ate a great deal, yet castigated herself for not being able to start another diet (Mode One). When she finally did "surrender to the struggle to lose weight," she'd choose a rigorous diet so she could see quick results (Mode Four). While dieting, Phyllis would feel testy and watch with envy those friends who were "naturally thin" (Mode Five). One friend even ended the friendship after Phyllis made a cutting remark.

Phyllis considered all of this angst part of what she had to do to lose weight. When she reached her goal, she felt at ease for a while, "but deep down inside I knew it wouldn't last. It never has" (Mode Seven). This sense of foreboding made failure even more depressing: "I'd struggled. Then I had to watch myself put it all back on, plus a few pounds. It made me bang the walls and scream. I always felt I was being cheated after suffering so much to be good. And I hated myself" (Mode Four and Mode Six).

At this point, Phyllis would think about going on a diet again (Mode One) and wait until an approaching class reunion or wedding motivated her to seek another magic formula (Mode Two). Observe, however, that no matter where she was in the process—weight up or down, spirits up or down—Phyllis was still in a diet mode.

Certainly, devoting so much energy to yo-yo dieting—the "rhythm method of girth control," as one patient calls it—is not a psychologically healthy way to live. But even though many dieters realize the emotional pitfalls, there are also motivations that perpetuate the modes.

A major factor is that physical appearance is so tied to self-esteem, particularly for women. A recent study at the Duke University Medical Center in Durham, North Carolina—the first study ever to look at the psychological impact of weight—found that mildly obese women exhibited lower self-esteem than morbidly obese men who were considerably heavier. The women also reported a more negative impact on their sex life, suggesting that esteem and sex "are more vulnerable areas for women, regardless of their weight."

The desire to be thin also creates an all-or-nothing mindset, so that even partial victories—a loss of 10 pounds instead of the desired 35, for example—are considered failures. Yet, a 10-pound loss can have a real impact on our quality of life, self-esteem, interest in sex, and energy levels. Rather than being encouraged by these improvements, the message of the diet modes—"Not good enough, you failed again"—prevails.

Physiology and the Diet Mentality

Psychology is not the only force that perpetuates the diet modes. There are also physiological factors at work that make weight loss difficult and strengthen diet thinking. Scientists at Rockefeller University in New York City recently concluded a ten-year study that confirmed what dieters have long suspected: As you lose weight, your body implements a complex system designed to return you to your original weight.

Your metabolism slows down so that you burn calories more slowly and less efficiently than before. With significant weight loss, the metabolism slows further, because the brain perceives that you are starving and tries to protect you from losing food stores. At one point in our evolution, the ability of the brain to do this was certainly an advantage; unfortunately, this is less true today.

In the Rockefeller study, the metabolism of dieting subjects became 10 to 15 percent slower than normal. This was true of all the dieters, whether they were overweight or of normal weight. The altered metabolism remains even after you have lost weight, so you can only maintain the weight loss by taking in fewer calories. If you go back to your old eating habits, weight comes on quickly, since your body is now burning calories more slowly.

If you don't know how to adapt successfully, you experience failure. You feel depressed and trapped as physiology and psychology work together to imprison you in the diet mentality.

How the Medications Help

Even though it may seem that body and mind are working against you, you don't have to let that be true. And here is where the medications—fenfluramine and phentermine—make such a powerful difference. Let's take a look at what happens.

On the psychological front, the drugs crash through the diet mentality. By giving your brain the simple message that you are full, they produce the following changes:

- You understand that you don't need willpower in order to lose weight, so there's no need to procrastinate about starting.

- You eat less with little effort, so you don't have to pretend to yourself that you're eating less than you really are.

- You see weight coming off rapidly, so you don't need to rely on a diet that makes you suffer.

- You do not feel deprived, so you have no reason to envy those who seemingly eat less without a sense of deprivation.

- You gain control over how much you eat, so you don't have to fear going back to your old eating habits.

Finally, you realize that, no matter what the Rockefeller University scientists discovered, you have the power to keep weight off if you take appropriate steps. Thanks to the medications, you are no longer tortured by a post-weight-loss sense of deprivation that causes you to eat more. You can persist in your new eating habits and continue to upgrade your level of physical activity.

By eating wisely, you maintain lower caloric intake. By exercising, you increase muscle mass and burn more calories. These measures thwart the body's natural efforts to return to its previous weight. Gradually, the struggle ceases, and your escape from the diet mode is complete. There may be setbacks along the way, but you can maintain the escape, with or without the drugs, depending on various factors I will discuss later on.

The psychological effects of abandoning the diet modes can be profound, with changes in self-image being among the most notable. One of my patients, for example, always thought of herself as "Gwen Smythe, fat woman." "That was it," she said. "There was nothing else about me that counted."

Although Gwen's husband was deeply in love with her, and always said that he found her attractive, Gwen didn't feel that way about herself. Everything that her husband praised—her skills in raising the children, her ability as an artist, her easy way of attracting friends who depended on her—took a back seat to the fact that she was overweight.

"Wherever we went, I was sure that the only thing people noticed about me was my weight. I even thought that men wanted to be my friends because they thought of me as motherly and women because they saw me as unthreatening. My weight kept me from getting an accurate picture of myself."

As the medications did their work, and Gwen abandoned her diet mentality, she liked the new body she saw in the mirror. But even more important, she was able to appreciate her own positive qualities because the "fat woman" had totally disappeared. The new image in the mirror, which Gwen knew was going to be a permanent one, triggered self-appreciation of her familiar qualities: mother, artist, loving wife, good friend, and loyal confidante. In short, for the first time, Gwen was able to view herself as a total human being.

Tim Baker, an oil company executive, saw himself as out of control when it came to weight. A yo-yo dieter for decades, he decided to escape the diet mentality by resolving not to diet anymore. "My new philosophy was: 'Hey, I'm heavy, so what? If it doesn't bother me, it shouldn't bother you.' " But denial turned out to be a diet mode in itself, since Tim resented having to think of himself as the kind of person who would give up on anything.

"It doesn't bother me" lasted about four months. No matter how much he pretended to himself, Tim imagined that his new supervisor—a man who had just been hired by the company—was disturbed by his appearance. "I heard that some people in the department were being shifted to another unit and I was certain that I was going to be one of them because this guy always looked at me strangely. Even though nothing happened, I still felt uneasy around him."

That was when Tim dropped the mask of not caring and came to see me. He was thrilled with the weight loss he achieved. But just as important, the medications gave him what he really needed to validate his self-image: a sense of control over his own body.

"I always wondered how someone like me, who has no trouble making tough decisions, meeting hectic schedules, or managing difficult people, could get defeated by a plate of food. It was a joke, like I had a chink in my armor or something. Now I feel as if my head is on straight. The joke is over."

Vestiges of the Diet Mentality

There are some patients who, for one reason or another, cling to the diet modes. They can see the weight coming off, they lose their food obsessions, but instead of enjoying a sense of liberation, they feel disquieted. They suspect that instead of being in charge of their own destiny, they are only ceding control to the drugs—an idea they find unacceptable. In response, they remain overweight or subconsciously set out to gain weight back.

Usually the people who fit this pattern have long histories of failed dieting. After being abandoned by the medical community, and not succeeding with commercial diet enterprises, they conclude that theirs is a personal struggle that can only be carried on without help from others. They become Spartan soldiers in the war against weight.

This was the philosophy of Cecelia Randall, a retail store owner, who had tried one approach after another, including therapy. Her psychologist referred her to me, and after evaluating Cecelia, I prescribed fenfluramine and phentermine. When I saw her a month later, she was annoyed and agitated and, despite her weight loss, told me right out that the pills didn't work for her. "I took them and I didn't like them. Besides, I take too many other pills."

Cecelia was on medication for hypertension and diabetes, two conditions directly related to her weight. But although she accepted the idea that these conditions were chronic and needed medication, she resisted the notion that obesity had to be treated the same way. Finally, she admitted that she preferred to achieve her weight goals without the use of the drugs. "I'll take them to get over the times when dieting and exercise don't work. But otherwise, no. I've learned to live with being hungry, and that's just the way it is for me."

For Cecelia, being on the medications was a sign of weakness. She had mentally resolved to no longer trust any form of assistance, even though this new discovery was clearly working. Such contradictory behavior is what can happen to people after they have been buffeted by too many trips through the diet mill.

I told Cecelia it was natural for individuals to want to have the final say over their bodies. That's why so many people resist taking medications for depression, for example, even when they are clearly suffering. But patients with depression can be victims of a chemical imbalance, just as overweight people may be. Is it realistic, I asked, to resist correcting a medical problem of any sort simply to maintain a sense of mastery?

I urge individuals who cling to the diet mode to think about whether their goal is to lose weight or to maintain a philosophy. If weight loss is what is wanted, these drugs will help to accomplish that goal. Generally, a discussion like this one persuades people to at least try the drugs for a longer period of time. This is what happened to Cecelia, who eventually dropped her opposition to the drugs and now regards them as one of the best things that ever happened to her.

Another reason for resisting the medications is that losing your food obsessions—and knowing they won't come back—can actually be traumatic. If you're accustomed to reaching for food in an emotionally trying situation, and you no longer get that urge, you may feel as if part of you has been snatched away. It's scary to have to give up an emotional crutch that's been soothing, but it can help to know that the crutch you depended on is hollow. By accepting its loss, you may be able to pay attention to deeper problems.

Cecelia, for example, found that she most often needed food after arguing with her ex-husband, who was also a part-owner of her retail business. For her, food obsessions were more comfortable than allowing her full range of feelings about this domineering man to surface.

After she agreed to take the medications I offered, Cecelia also decided to continue working with the therapist who had referred her to me. With the obsessions gone, she found she was able to make great progress in dealing with other problem areas of her life.

Testing the Power of Success

Another vestige of the diet mentality is the need of some people to test the waters of "normal" eating as soon as they've lost weight. Although it hasn't been difficult for them to adopt new nutritional patterns, they start stocking up the refrigerator with foods they know spell trouble—and, quite quickly, trouble follows.

Sometimes, the individuals who do this have been ideal patients, following my instructions faithfully, developing their own food plans, and keeping all of their appointments. But after reaching their goal, I may not hear from them for six months or even longer. When they do come back, they are usually bashful and repentant because they have put the weight back on.

Since obesity is a chronic condition, earlier patterns of behavior can be quite compelling; there is no reason to blame oneself for giving in. The important thing is to start the program again and to realize that obesity won't just go away. It needs to be managed every single day of the year. By being aware of when you stop managing—skipping the medication for a day or two, cutting back on exercise, increasing trips to fast-food restaurants—you can make the appropriate effort to get back into control.

There is another self-defeating approach that some patients take after weight loss. They abruptly stop the medications without checking with me. This is like pulling the plug on the entire program because, for many, food obsessions, poor eating habits, and sedentary ways are likely to return. Why do people pursue such a course? I believe there is a strong need to believe the weight problem has been solved, once and for all, even though I have explained many times that this is impossible.

"Why is this happening to me when I was cured?" one patient asked. This man first came to see me because he wanted to lose what he called his "postdivorce flab." He did wonderfully on the medications and then I didn't see him for almost a year.

He showed up late one winter afternoon, flab restored, and wondering what had happened to his "cure." My patient, who was quite intelligent, didn't want to accept the chronicity of his condition. "I guess I was like an alcoholic, falling off the wagon," he told me, after we discussed the matter.

As with any long-term situation, it may take time before acceptance is reached. This particular patient had to "fall off the wagon" several times until he realized that he had to continue the program. Now he keeps in touch with me every month, enjoys the eating system he developed, and is determined to keep on exercising. He is happy for his second chances and feels he may finally be kicking the diet mindset. If so, that would be the best "cure" of all.

Treatment Forever?

Since continuing to take the medications can be an issue, let me say that some patients are able to maintain goal weight without the drugs, but others are not. Who will succeed, of course, only becomes apparent over time, so my general approach is as follows:

- After six months or so on the program, I look at several factors. How much weight has this person lost? Is he or she tolerating the medications well? Is the individual eating sensibly and exercising regularly?
- If there has been a significant weight loss—15 percent of body weight, for example—and programmatic participation is strong, I begin to gradually eliminate the medications. This can be done by having the patient take only one of the medications, alternating the medications, or reducing dosages of both medications.
- During this process, I watch very carefully, because the tendency to regain weight without the drugs may be strong. The people who do best without the drugs are those who observe dietary changes rigorously and exercise with the same degree of dedication. Interestingly, such people will often say that they no longer feel hungry, even off the medications, indicating to my mind that the drugs may have a long-term effect on the brain chemistry of certain individuals.

Even with the best of intentions, however, the general pattern is for weight to be regained at some point. My experience is that only a small percentage of people can keep the weight off without intermittent use of the drugs. I call this intermittent use "pulsing." If I observe that a person has gained 10 pounds, I put him or her back on the medications for several months until the weight is lost again. Some people have to be "pulsed" quite often. Others can go for long periods of time without gaining any weight.

The point is, you can't know for sure when weight gain is going to occur, or even if it's going to occur. But you have to prepare yourself for this formidable enemy by regarding the medications as a lifetime aid. There is no reason to feel bad about needing periodic assistance. It is just a fact, pure and simple.

In seven months, Nicole Tremont, a physical therapist, achieved her goal of losing 45 pounds. Two months later, I had Nicole gradually stop using the drugs to see what would happen. Within six months, she had put on 10 pounds.

Nicole was quite upset, but I was quick to point out that the weight gain did not imply any failure on her part. Best not to think in terms of failure at all, since that is the diet mentality. Instead, Nicole had to view the drugs, rather neutrally, as a tool that was available to her.

She went back on the medications, lost the 10 pounds, and continued the drugs for one month after that. Since that time, a year ago, Nicole has not gained any weight, but she understands that she might at some time in the future. She isn't worried; she doesn't test herself by eating too much or exercising too little; she doesn't put herself through the grinding mill of the diet modes. She is simply prepared to be "pulsed" if the need arises.

I have found that a small percentage of my patients are not in their overweight state when they initially come to see me. Through their own efforts—some using low-calorie diets, some combining dieting with exercise—they have succeeded in reaching their weight-loss goals. But they see their weight start to creep back once they exhaust their willpower to remain food-deprived. They, too, want to escape the diet mentality and are eager to explore the use of medications to control their chronic condition. After taking a complete history, as I do with all my patients, and understanding that they are motivated to follow through with all aspects of my program, I start pulsing them in the same way as I do with patients who have lost weight using the medications.

There is a wonderful freedom that comes when one stops thinking like a dieter. Even if some weight comes back, it will be temporary if you don't succumb to the diet mentality, because it's so easy to take steps to correct the situation. And if there's one thing those troubling diet modes can't survive, it's a sensible attitude.

CHAPTER NINE

Why More and More Physicians Are Believers

For a good part of each year, my schedule includes making early-morning rounds at Manhattan's Bellevue Hospital with a group of ten or so medical residents. It is here, with the sick and dying patients in front of us, that I'm best able to point out the far-reaching effects of obesity on health.

Invariably, the experience turns out to be an eye-opener for these young men and women. For four years, they've been reading textbooks, attending lectures, and doing laboratory work. But now, for the first time, they see patients and treat illness on a daily basis. Because they are on the firing line, they must respond to the complex symptoms that acute care inevitably involves.

Over and over, my residents witness the devastating effects of obesity, yet somehow they continue to regard the ailment as it was presented to them in medical school—as simply a risk factor for certain diseases, such as heart disease, diabetes, and hypertension. With this instruction, it's not surprising that we have produced yet another generation of physicians who believe that all a person has to do to lose weight is switch to a low-fat diet, eat less, and exercise three times a week.

I've found the newer generation of physicians and residents to be extremely caring and sensitive individuals. However, when it comes to obesity, like most Americans, they still have a blind spot. I make it a point to ask them what they think about the meaning of obesity. When I do, I usually get responses like the following:

- "When a patient is overweight, I find it difficult to listen to the heart and lungs with a stethoscope."
- "A fatty abdomen is harder to examine. You can't feel for masses through the layers of fat."
- "I've observed that laparoscopic surgery is more difficult because the surgeon has to go through thick layers of fat to get to organs like the gallbladder."
- "Fat people are usually in poor physical shape so they don't recover from surgery as well."
- "There are many wound-healing problems because of the decreased vascularity of fat."

Notice the emphasis here on the technological aspects of medicine—the examination, the surgery, the wound care— and also on the problems that too much weight presents for the physician rather than the patient.

Medical education, instead of being instructive, fails to provide young doctors with the results of current research about excess weight. So, today's physicians, like the rest of the population, rely on the media for most of their information about obesity studies.

Study after study has found physiological and biochemical evidence that obesity is a complex disorder of energy metabolism. Some forms of obesity have a genetic cause, as confirmed by the recent discovery of the *ob* gene that appears to signal the brain to regulate weight (see Chapter 11). The evidence points to the conclusion that most people have little control over their weight, which is why pounds can be kept off only by frantically monitoring every morsel of food.

By now, I've gotten used to the fact that many physicians remain stubbornly unaware of the new research. Without the appropriate medical school education, it's difficult for doctors to have their consciousness raised. Still, it frustrates me that many new doctors have the same biases that existed twenty years ago, and I've taken it upon myself to try to educate the residents whenever I can. I have them analyze their work with overweight patients, so they come to realize how difficult losing weight can be and how much the medications can help.

Dr. John Reynolds, a resident in internal medicine, was treating Tiffany Burke, an outpatient in the hospital clinic who suffered from diabetes. At 50 pounds above her ideal weight, Tiffany badly needed to lose weight to get her diabetes under control. After watching John examine Tiffany, I said I thought she could benefit from medications, and I explained the way that fenfluramine and phentermine work. Tiffany's chart showed that she had been overweight all of her life, and the diabetes, which had been discovered five months earlier, posed a serious threat.

John looked at me skeptically when I offered him a copy of an article by Dr. Michael Weintraub about his research on the drugs. "Tiffany's just a glutton who needs to exercise more," he told me. "I'm going to recommend an increase in her dose of insulin and get her to begin walking a few times a week. That should be easy enough for her to do."

As he closed the file, I looked at John's 6'4" frame. "Not an inch of fat on him," I thought. I remembered John telling me how he lifted weights several times a week and ran every day, despite his long shifts as a resident. "Exercise keeps me going," he had said.

To John, it seemed natural enough to want to exercise. He had not reckoned on how daunting exercising can be to a person like Tiffany who had never done much of it. I suggested that losing some weight on the medication can motivate a person to start exercising, but John said he didn't see why a patient would need a "crutch." "Besides," he went on, "I thought the main issue here was the diabetes."

I was going to ask John whether he thought insulin was a "crutch," too, but after all, Tiffany was his patient. I held my tongue.

When John saw Tiffany a month later, she told him she had started a walking program, but she hadn't lost any weight. This seemed incredible to John, and I think he questioned Tiffany's veracity, but she'd been keeping a diary of where she walked and for how long. She felt frustrated by her failure, and she told John that her food urges seemed to be growing stronger.

"She must be eating too much or not eating the right kinds of foods," John told me. He took down a careful record of Tiffany's eating patterns and then referred her to a nutritionist who specialized in diabetes. I could see that diabetes was still the problem uppermost on John's mind.

The nutritionist prepared an eating plan for Tiffany; she followed it and began to lose weight. As the months went by, John reported the pounds lost to me with a look of triumph on his face. "I knew it was just a question of diet," he said.

But soon after Tiffany took off all the weight she needed to lose, the pounds began to come back on. I explained that dieting had caused Tiffany's metabolism to slow down, so adding even a bit more food to her daily regimen caused her to regain weight. I told John how I "pulsed" the medications to keep patients from regaining weight, but I could see he really wasn't listening.

Rather than opening himself up to new information, John was still reviewing the "medical" possibilities. "Perhaps she has a thyroid condition that we haven't picked up," he said. "I'll arrange for her to see a specialist and have some more sensitive tests done."

Tiffany's tests came back negative, a result that didn't surprise me, but by this time Tiffany herself was becoming annoyed at John. "She told me that she didn't know why she had to waste her time with all this," John reported to me. "She said she was coming to the point where she'd rather die than have to try one more doctor or one more diet."

Tiffany's mental attitude had just about convinced John that she needed to see a psychiatrist. "Maybe there's some emotional reason for her weight," he said. "Perhaps she was molested as a child. Or maybe she has a death wish."

He picked up the phone to consult with the psychiatry department, then slowly put it down again. "The fact is, Steve," he said, "I'm feeling pretty frustrated myself. I can't seem to help this lady, so maybe that's why I'm annoyed with her. But I just can't figure out why a person wouldn't want to lose weight when their health is involved."

It was a matter of "can't" rather than not wanting to, I said. We wouldn't expect a patient to cure any other condition by willpower, so why feel that way about someone's weight? For the first time, I could see that the concept of obesity as a disease was making an impression, but John seemed to fight it off.

"There *are* people who lose weight and keep it off," he insisted. "How do you explain them?"

It turned out that John was talking about the author of a best-selling book who had lost weight through extreme deprivation, including a low-calorie liquid diet. In this particular "success story," the author's family locked up food to keep it away from her, and continued to do so even after she lost weight.

I asked John if he would recommend that his patients live this way. I also pointed out that we didn't know whether the author would be any more successful at maintaining her weight loss than Tiffany Burke had been.

"All right," John said, "but what about those celebrities who lose weight?"

The livelihood of celebrities depends on their size and shape, I countered. They have unlimited resources at their disposal to keep weight under control—cooks to prepare special foods, personal fitness trainers to work with them four hours a day, cosmetic surgery, liposuction, and other medical procedures.

As for the "diet gurus" who lose weight and then make a career out of preaching to others, they are Big Business. The

Diet Industry generates more than $33 billion annually, and in order to keep a piece of the pie, a guru has to stay thin. Doctors can't compare their patients to these people, and certainly patients shouldn't compare themselves to them either.

In the real world, weight loss is maintained in only 5 percent of cases. If a treatment modality had a failure rate of 95 percent, I asked John, wouldn't you want to explore other options? "Twenty years from now," I concluded, "scientists will look back on our approach to weight loss as barbaric. But we can start to make changes right now."

I invited John to come to my office and talk with patients about the effects produced by phentermine and fenfluramine. By reviewing the clinical data in the files—which was indisputable—he became a convert. John later gave Tiffany a copy of the Weintraub study and offered her an alternative. He suggested that she consult with a physician who treated obesity with phentermine and fenfluramine.

Tiffany later called John to thank him. She took off the 50 pounds she had to lose, continued her walking program, and added other exercise as well. Today, Tiffany feels confident about her ability to keep her weight under control without a sense of struggle and deprivation. If she needs "help" from drugs, so be it. That's certainly a whole lot better than constantly feeling angry at herself—and her physician.

John is pleased with the treatment of Tiffany's diabetes and also with the treatment of her weight problem. He realizes now that he was attacking two conditions, not one.

As the efficiency of the drugs becomes better known, more physicians will no doubt undergo a change in attitude like John's. As increasing numbers of patients have the drugs prescribed for them, and continue to achieve dramatic results, the physiological causes of obesity will become apparent. This, in turn, will make it even more acceptable to prescribe drugs for this medical condition. The cycle, we hope, will be similar to the way that the medication Prozac (fluoxetine) impacted on our acceptance of depression as a disease with biological components.

Recently, a panel of experts from the Institutes of Medicine concluded that obesity should be regarded not as a cosmetic problem but as "an important chronic, degenerative disease that debilitates individuals and kills prematurely." The panel also urged health professionals to administer anti-obesity drugs so they are "treated similarly to those used for the treatment of other medical problems, such as hypertension." The panel's conclusions demonstrate a distinct acceptance of the value of current anti-obesity medications. And the Food and Drug Administration (FDA), aware of the $100 billion in health-care costs caused by obesity, is speeding the way for approval of new medications.

Currently, FDA regulations require drug companies to test anti-obesity drugs on human subjects for two years and to prove that the drugs not only help in weight loss but also lower the risk for heart disease, diabetes, hypertension, and other obesity-related conditions. Under proposed new guidelines, the drugs will only have to be tested for one year, with weight loss the sole criterion for success. In addition, there will be a follow-up year of testing to determine the safety of the drugs.

"The tide is certainly turning in regard to the pharmacological treatment of overweight people," says Glenn Braunstein, M.D., chairman of the department of medicine at Cedars-Sinai Medical Center, professor of medicine at the University of California/Los Angeles, and head of the medical committee advising the FDA on obesity drugs.

Braunstein believes that thirty years of negative attitudes

toward obesity medication, generated by the amphetamine-based drugs, are finally changing. As physicians increasingly realize that the new medications work through the serotonergic system of the brain, they are becoming much more comfortable about prescribing them.

The medical profession still has work to do to both educate young doctors about the drugs and to take back control of weight treatment from the diet industry. But, there are now a growing number of physicians who are doing just that. I predict that within two years, most physicians in the United States will be prescribing these drugs. Currently, however, there are still many doctors unfamiliar with the medications and appropriate treatments for obesity. That's why it's important for you to know how to select a doctor who can help you, a subject I'll discuss next.

CHAPTER TEN

Finding the Help You Need

Before undertaking the search for a qualified physician, you'll need to determine your own readiness to commit to a medically supervised treatment program. Are you motivated enough to follow through with a comprehensive program that includes the use of medications? To find out, ask yourself these questions:

• *Do I fully accept the fact that my weight is threatening my health?* If you already have a cardiac condition, diabetes, arthritis, hypertension, or some other weight-related problem, do you understand the importance of losing weight and keeping it off?

• *Is my weight affecting my self-image?* If your weight makes you feel down on yourself, unattractive, and uncertain about achieving career or social goals, weight loss can provide a psychological makeover—and whether you realize it or not, your motivation to get thinner is already in place.

• *Is my weight interfering with my lifestyle?* If you can't do the things you want to do—learn a new skill, take up a sport, or even play ball with children or grandchildren—you are missing too much. Losing weight can open locked doors. There is plenty here to draw on to find motivation.

• *Is my weight messing up my family life?* If your weight has become an issue, if you feel you're being nagged constantly and your loved ones fear for your health, weight loss can do more good than a family therapist. Motivation can emerge from viewing weight loss as therapeutic.

• *Have I accepted the fact that excessive weight is a chronic medical condition requiring a lifetime of management?* If you have been on the psychologically damaging weight loss–weight gain roller coaster, you must realize that excessive weight is not something that can be "cured" but rather it needs to be treated and managed with the help of your physician.

Once you decide that losing weight and keeping it off is a priority, and not just a casual thought, half of the battle is won. No matter how many times you have fought this particular war in the past, this time, with medication on your side, you can achieve victory.

Locating a Physician

As I noted earlier, not all physicians in the United States today are using fenfluramine and phentermine. I believe that familiarity with the medications and a willingness to prescribe them should be among your criteria in selecting a physician. This is because I have observed, over and over again, the power of these drugs.

You may not have to look any farther than your primary-care physician. Generally, this is the doctor who knows you and your problems the best. But if you think your primary physician has little interest in weight loss and views excessive weight as a character flaw, tends to downplay its seriousness, or looks upon losing weight as something that can be easily done, you'd be well advised to find another doctor. Don't be embarrassed to ask your primary physician for a referral to a physician who has experience in treating obesity and is currently using phentermine and fenfluramine with his or her patients.

About 60 percent of the obesity specialists who comprise the membership of the American Society of Bariatric Physicians prescribe medications as a part of their comprehensive program. A bariatric physician is a medical doctor who has a special interest in the study and treatment of obese patients and their associated conditions. For a list of member physicians in your area, contact The American Society of Bariatric Physicians, 5600 South Quebec, Suite 109A, Englewood, CO; tel. 303-779-4833.

Another option is to ask for a referral from friends or relatives who have successfully lost weight using medications. As more and more people successfully manage their weight with the use of these drugs, referrals will become more frequent.

Local hospitals and medical centers are also good sources of physician referrals. Be sure to state your basic qualification: a physician with a great deal of experience in helping people lose weight with the medications. It may be necessary for the person assisting you in your search to ask around in the hospital, rather than simply read names off a roster. Don't hesitate to ask for this type of research.

For a good family practitioner or internist, you can contact your county medical society. If you can't find a physician who already uses the phentermine and fenfluramine, you should, at the very least, look for someone who is willing to review the material in this book and the medical literature. It's been my experience that responsive physicians, rather than resenting new information from patients, welcome the opportunity to expand the scope of their practice. It's up to the doctor, of course, to decide whether to proceed. But it may be up to you to broach the subject. If you believe that the drugs can help your weight-loss efforts, then speak up. If you have found the right doctor, he or she will at least be willing to listen.

Before you set up an appointment with a physician, do some checking on your own. Nearly all libraries have directories that can give you information about educational background, hospital affiliation, and other pertinent physician credentials.

Be Prepared

Organize to get the most out of your first visit. Take along the special tear-out section at the back of this book containing my letter to your physician and handy medical references concerning the use of medications in treating obesity. Also, jot down your weight-loss history so that you can discuss it with the physician. Don't overlook the failures; these will play an important role in future planning. Make a list of all the drugs you are currently taking, as the doctor will need this information.

Also list the questions you'll want to discuss, such as:

- How do you treat patients with fenfluramine and phentermine?
- Do you prescribe the medications for long-term use?

Arrive at the doctor's office fully prepared to discuss your medical condition. When you're called in for your appointment, the doctor will probably take a complete medical history before examining you. A doctor who is savvy about weight control will focus on your weight-loss history as well. He or she will also ask about other people in your family who are overweight, looking for a possible genetic connection. The doctor may investigate the possibility of thyroid disease or adrenal gland disorder.

Don't hesitate to ask your physician about complications associated with obesity, such as sleep apnea, hypertension, arthritis, or diabetes. Take your time in talking about your problem. An appropriate doctor will listen carefully, ask significant questions—such as why you think other methods of weight loss did not work in the past—and evaluate your level of motivation. What you need to do is observe the doctor just as carefully. Do you have the feeling of being rushed?

Surveys show that many doctors do not listen enough. In a 1984 analysis of seventy-four medical interviews, doctors interrupted their patients, on average, eighteen seconds after they had begun to speak, halting the flow of information and imposing their own ideas. With weight loss, a doctor must understand where you have been in the past and what you hope to accomplish now. That requires not only listening but also a sympathetic spirit.

Just as a doctor should be respectful of the patient's concerns, the patient needs to have an appropriate sense of the value of the doctor's time. Physicians are busy today—and a good physician is going to have a large practice—so zero in with your pertinent questions.

A physician has to convey a feeling of understanding and support. Empathy is a difficult quality to evaluate rationally, but most of us know when it's missing. A good physician will demonstrate empathy not only by asking about you, but by explaining his or her own background in obesity, philosophy, and program. Now it's your turn to listen. If a doctor is judgmental about past failures, tells you that weight loss is easy enough to accomplish with willpower, hands you a piece of paper with a diet on it, or refuses to discuss medications as an option, you need to look elsewhere.

A partnership must be established between you and the physician and you should view it as such. He or she should expect you to be involved in food planning, exercise development, and decision making. A good weight-loss physician will require your active participation for a successful outcome.

Getting On Schedule

Once you decide to work with a physician, make sure you understand how matters will proceed. First, you should know what tests the doctor will be performing and when the results will be shared with you.

Before starting the medications, expect the doctor to review possible side effects with you. You should also get some idea of how long you can expect side effects to last and what you can do to diminish them.

You should also receive specific instructions as to when to take the drugs and when to come in for follow-up visits. For example, I will see patients as frequently as every two weeks when initiating a medication program and there are complicating issues involved such as hypertension. Others, who are doing much better, may come to see me every two months. The bottom line is that this is an individualized approach that can't be regimented; your physician will need to see you as often as is necessary to treat your medical condition.

It's also important for the physician to make telephone time available to answer questions. A doctor who understands weight loss will readily do this. Some doctors have a specific phone hour. Others will simply return phone calls. You should be able to get an idea of how long it will take to have your call returned and try to be as specific as possible when you do speak.

Dealing with Your Insurance Coverage

As I've already mentioned, the direct economic costs of not treating obesity effectively are currently estimated to be over $40 billion nationwide. Researchers peg this amount to represent almost 6 percent of all medical costs in the United States.

It is eminently clear that obesity is a health issue that must be addressed. By seeking medical treatment for obesity from your physician, you are certainly taking a positive step. Also taking similar positive steps are some medical insurance companies that have wisely agreed to reimburse patients for obesity treatment, covering both physician visits and medications. By reducing the incidence of obesity, these companies have surely seen a drop in their payments for obesity-related diseases such as hypertension, sleep apnea, and diabetes. In light of this, I envision a time soon when the necessity for medical treatment of obesity will become more obvious to every insurance company and these companies will also institute similar programs.

The good news is that more and more companies are reimbursing the primary diagnosis of obesity. Check your own policy to see if you are covered. If you are not, have your physician write a letter on your behalf justifying your treatment to the medical director of your insurance company. Also, photocopy or cut out the special section at the end of the book entitled **For Your Physician.**

If obesity as a medical diagnosis is not covered under your plan, it is quite possible that an alternative diagnosis that you have, such as hypertension, diabetes, sleep apnea disorder, degenerative arthritis, or hiatal hernia, is covered by your policy.

As the medical community begins to embrace the new therapeutic approach to treating obesity, data will be presented to the insurance companies and they, too, will accept obesity as a medical diagnosis and offer full coverage for its treatment and management.

Counting on Family and Friends

Generally speaking, people who want to lose weight can use all the assistance they can get. Often, that means seeking the support of family and friends. But sometimes—especially if you've attempted many times to lose weight in the past—your support system may not be prepared for yet another go-round. "My family simply doesn't want to hear about my trying to lose weight again," a patient once said in a discouraged tone.

This woman's husband felt that he had been "through the

mill" too often. "Every time she diets, it's like preparing for a war I know she's going to lose," he confided to me after his wife had left the room. "I'd rather see her overweight than disappointed one more time."

If you suspect that your family may be feeling this way, it's important to explain the qualitative difference that fenfluramine and phentermine represent. Often, what upsets families is the way that weight-loss struggles can make a person short-tempered, irritable, and just plain hungry all the time. With the medications, none of this happens, so life is a whole lot easier for everyone concerned.

It will also reassure your family to know exactly how the drugs work. They should understand that when you are on the medications, you will feel full, satisfied, and comfortable around food. This time, they will not have to nag, coddle, or duck for cover when you become angry at yourself. In short, they will not be entering a war zone simply because you have decided to lose weight.

It is also important to make your family aware of how helpful they can be. Sometimes the atmosphere surrounding weight loss becomes so emotional that families either feel left out or stretched too thin. That's why it's a good idea to be as direct and specific as possible.

Here are some of the suggestions my patients have found useful and that you can adapt to your own situation:

- *Encourage me to stick to my medication schedule.* Remind me that any side effects will pass. Don't let me stop taking the medications because I think I have lost enough weight.
- *Help me to develop and follow an eating plan.* Try to share my new enthusiasm for nutrition. Understand that I am not diet-

ing, but trying to change my way of eating. Don't sabotage me by preparing foods I've decided to avoid or suggesting that we go out to buffet restaurants.

• *Remind me to make time for exercise.* If I've always been a nonexerciser, review options with me. Perhaps there's something you enjoy doing that we can share. If I need an exercise buddy, can I count on you?

• *Support me through setbacks.* If I get mad at myself for overeating, remind me that tomorrow is another day. If I neglect the medications, suggest that I make an appointment with my doctor. Help me get back on track by showing that my weight loss is important to you.

If there is someone else in your family who needs to lose weight, encourage that person to take part in the program with you. In weight loss, a partnership can be a powerful combination.

When Support Is Lacking

Unfortunately, sometimes people who should be your supporters can sabotage you in subtle—and not so subtle—ways. For example, the "best friend" of one of my patients suggested that they go on a cruise together shortly after my patient had announced his resolve to avoid situations that encouraged him to overeat. When my patient recommended another kind of trip, the friend suddenly became too busy at work to go anyplace at all.

A supportive person will generally validate your reasons for wanting to lose weight, want to learn about the medications,

x

and demonstrate enthusiasm for your new eating and exercise plans. Nonsupportive people will, consciously or unconsciously, subvert your game plan by asking questions like these: "Why take drugs when losing weight is just a matter of willpower?" "Why does everyone in this family have to change their eating habits just because you're on another diet?" "Why can't you stop the medications now? I think you've lost enough weight."

Obviously, when you hear too many "why" questions and too few "how can I help" offers, you know you need to look elsewhere for assistance. Better to talk regularly on the phone with a supportive friend than get into hassles with a nonsupportive family member.

Not getting support can be tough, but you need to remind yourself that you can succeed, even working on your own. Losing weight, getting healthier, looking better—these are your goals and they will improve your well-being. That's why you need to be personally committed to them, even though every single family member may not be. Remember, too, that attitudes can change when a relative observes your own level of commitment. Finally, is it always a good idea to involve family and friends in your plans? Not necessarily. Some people, I've found, would rather keep their weight-loss efforts to themselves.

No matter what you decide, remember that the medications can provide a level of control that hasn't been available before. But these drugs—rather than being the alpha and omega of what can be accomplished pharmacologically—are really just the beginning.

CHAPTER ELEVEN

The Next Wave

Even with the tremendous success of phentermine and fen-fluramine, we are just at the dawn of a new era in the treatment of obesity. In laboratories around the world, scientists are working to develop new medications. These medications, when combined with wholesome eating and regular exercise, will greatly simplify the process of losing excess pounds and keeping them off.

"Pharmacology is the wave of the future in treating obesity," says Richard Atkinson, M.D., president of the American Society for Clinical Nutrition and a professor of medicine and nutritional science at the University of Wisconsin, Madison. "It's been adequately demonstrated that people are not going to change their eating behavior through diet, exercise, and behavior modification alone," Atkinson states. "Therefore, we are going to have to rely more heavily on medications."

The number of obese Americans rose by 30 percent from

1980 to 1990, Atkinson points out, due mainly to decreased physical activity. The amount of exercise we get has diminished significantly, aided by inventions that encourage inactivity, such as VCRs and television remote controls.

But even as the number of people suffering from obesity grows, relatively little money is earmarked for obesity research. Each year, only $35 million is spent on finding ways to unlock its cause and develop treatments. Even with this relatively limited expenditure of funds, remarkable strides have been made. Let's talk about some of these advances.

The *ob* Gene

In 1994, Jeffrey Friedman, Ph.D., a molecular geneticist at The Rockefeller University in New York City, described how he discovered first in mice, and then in human beings, a gene that seems to be related to obesity. In research performed on mice, Friedman observed a connection between the gene and weight gain.

The *ob* gene, which is nearly identical in mouse and human, seems to be switched on in the fat tissue where it generates a hormone-like protein that is secreted by the fat cells into the bloodstream. Friedman theorizes that when the gene is working normally, it helps to regulate weight by sending the brain a hormonal message to stop eating. However, when the gene is mutated or damaged, it either fails to make the proper hormone or it creates an abnormal hormone. As a result, the brain does not receive the message and the individual gains weight.

Although it's too early to be certain, obesity experts suspect that gene mutations may account for extreme variations in weight—why one person is 20 pounds overweight and another person 100 pounds overweight, for example. Friedman and other biotechnological scientists hope to engineer genetically a protein that will help regulate the gene. In the future, obesity could be treated by taking cells from an obese person, genetically altering them in the laboratory, and then injecting them back into the patient. Ultimately, this approach—gene therapy —would put an end to obesity by changing basic genetic structure. Another possibility is the development of a safe drug that would alter genetic structure in the same manner as gene therapy. Here again, the end result would be to help overweight people lose weight without a sense of deprivation or hunger.

While all this sounds good in theory, it may be complicated to achieve. Gene experts suspect, for example, that rather than one gene directly controlling obesity, there may be as many as ten. In addition, there may be up to 1,000 different genes taking part in the overall process leading to weight loss. Another complication is that Friedman's experiments involved only mice, not human beings. It is possible that human beings, unlike mice, are not affected by mutations of the *ob* gene.

Pharmaceutical companies didn't think so, and they put unprecedented amounts of money in *ob* gene research. Amgen, Inc., a California-based biotechnology company, won a bidding war to develop Friedman's work and paid Rockefeller University $20 million, with $100 million to come if the company successfully developed a gene-altering drug. Should Amgen produce such a drug, experts say, the company will have cornered the market on obesity treatment.

Friedman's leptin, which was the first weight-regulating

gene discovered, adds to the ever-growing body of medical knowledge that obesity is a chronic medical condition requiring medical solutions. Unfortunately, leptin as the definitive link between appetite and weight has so far not lived up to its initial high expectations.

After extensively testing 275 subjects, geneticists at Thomas Jefferson University in Philadelphia concluded in early 1996 that the overweight patients in their study in fact had plenty of leptin circulating in their bodies—some had four times as much of the hormone than their slimmer counterparts. According to the researchers, the problem was that, although leptin is an important factor in how much food is eaten, the brain for some unknown reason fails to respond or otherwise act upon leptin's all-important "stop eating" message.

Scientists worldwide are continuing in their dogged pursuit of unraveling the secrets of obesity, with many research labs investigating why some people fail to react appropriately to leptin. Perhaps, as scientists at Millennium Pharmaceuticals in Cambridge, Massachusetts, announced, it's not leptin or its lack, but rather it's the leptin receptors that are faulty in some people. The leptin receptors that the Millennium researchers discovered are heavily concentrated in the ventricles of the brain and seem to receive the fullness message from leptin and pass it on to the brain. The actual cause of obesity, say the researchers, may be due to faulty leptin receptors—and not leptin—which prevent the chemical signal of fullness from ever reaching the brain.

To date, leptin-receptor research has been performed on mice, not humans, and whether there is actually something wrong with leptin receptors in obese humans still needs to be determined. Still, with the discovery of the elusive leptin receptor, scientists now hope that they'll be able to find out the receptor's complete role in regulating appetite and energy metabolism and eventually bring about change. Their ultimate aim will be to create drugs that specifically act on those receptors so the "stop eating" message gets through to the brain as it's supposed to. Still, creating medications that can effectively bring this about pose enormous difficulties which may take years to overcome.

This is all good news. With research ongoing and setbacks regularly counterbalanced by new biological discoveries affecting weight, parts of the puzzle are slowly being put together piece by piece. Jeffrey Friedman's leptin discovery was certainly a major breakthrough, and it still may yield practical results in the near future. Thanks to Friedman, the first important step was taken, and scientists are quickly proceeding to more advanced levels of research.

GLP-1

A newly discovered protein in the brain's hypothalamus called glucagon-like peptide-1, or GLP-1, is now thought to be a major player in controlling food intake. Scientists in England recently noted that test rats ate virtually nothing after being injected with GLP-1, yet they still appeared to be full, even tired, as if they'd eaten a large meal. Even for those rats that hadn't eaten in a day, the GLP-1 injection squelched their hunger and reduced their food intake by 95 percent.

Experts now think that GLP-1 may be the most potent natural appetite suppressant found in rats. As for humans, the British scientists who spearheaded the research are virtually positive that humans have it in their brains as well because it's been found in every species of vertebrate. This suggests that treatments used for animals will probably work for humans as well.

Again, I applaud this research because it hopefully will result in more options for physicians to treat those patients whose weight leaves them at increased risk for illness. As with earlier leptin and leptin-receptor research, only further experimentation will prove if GLP-1 is indeed a formidable player in appetite regulation. Researchers are now trying to see if leptin triggers production of GLP-1 in the brain.

The next step with GLP-1 is to develop a pill suitable for human testing, something that could take as little as two years. In theory, after swallowing the pill, the medication would eventually reach the brain, mimic GLP-1, and thereby cause a person to eat less.

Galanin/Neuropeptide Y

One area under investigation is the chemistry of the brain itself. For the past two decades, Sarah Leibowitz, Ph.D., an associate professor of behavioral neurobiology at The Rockefeller University, has been pursuing this line of inquiry. In the 1970s, she discovered that the paraventricular nucleus (PVN), a tiny portion of the hypothalamus, was the source of appetite control. Instead of being responsible only for releasing milk in lactating mothers, as had previously been thought, the PVN was the primary activator of eating and drinking behavior.

Further research showed that specific chemical stimulation of the PVN led to increased eating. Leibowitz discovered that two neuropeptides—small compounds formed by the union of two or more amino acids—regulate desires for specific types of foods. The neuropeptide Y (NPY) stimulates the appetite for carbohydrates and another neuropeptide, galanin, stimulates the appetite for fat-laden foods.

In Leibowitz's animal studies, irregularities in NPY and galanin often correspond to overeating. Animals that eat a lot of fat and gain weight, for example, have high levels of galanin in the PVN.

Dr. Leibowitz is looking into how levels of galanin can be controlled. Drugs that suppress the synthesis of the neuropeptides, she believes, would hold great promise for the treatment of obesity. "They would have the potential to be more potent than anything we have now." Currently, she says, two or three pharmaceutical companies are "close to coming up with something effective. Within a year or two, clinical trials will be started."

Dexfenfluramine

Trials have already been performed, both in the United States and abroad, on dexfenfluramine, a drug that many experts consider to be a more potent version of fenfluramine. Like fenfluramine, dexfenfluramine is not an amphetamine, and it has no addictive potential. It reduces appetite—particularly abnormal appetite for carbohydrates—by affecting the brain chemical serotonin.

In 1982, Richard Wurtman, M.D., and Judith Wurtman, Ph.D., researchers at the Massachusetts Institute of Technology in Cambridge, licensed the patent for dexfenfluramine from a French pharmaceutical company. They further developed the drug, which had been used successfully and has been approved in more than fifty countries other than the United States for over a decade.

Dexfenfluramine seems to affect weight loss without altering metabolic rate. In one study of severely obese women, the drug not only increased satiety, it also limited the decrease in metabolism that typically slows down weight loss. Dexfenfluramine has also been shown to be effective in treating hypertension and diabetes.

For the majority of patients, the side effects of dexfenfluramine are minor, well-tolerated, and short-lived. In one trial of 782 subjects, side effects, including fatigue, diarrhea, dry mouth, and increased urinary frequency, diminished or disappeared as time of use lengthened. There has been some controversial research, however. Primary pulmonary hypertension (PPH), a rare, yet potentially dangerous lung disorder, has recently been recognized and associated with appetite-suppressant drugs containing fenfluramine. The incidence of PPH is estimated to be as low as 18 cases per million to as high as 46 cases per million patients per year. To put this in perspective, this is close to the risk of death associated with the use of two common drugs, penicillin and oral contraceptives.

This recent data is based on European research, and it is unclear what dosages the patients were given, the length of time they were using the medication, or if they had other medical conditions or poor health habits—such as smoking —that may have affected their condition.

Unfortunately, there is no diagnostic procedure that can predict PPH. As a precautionary measure, I advise my patients using fenfluramine and dexfenfluramine to immediately report any unusual and persistent shortness of breath, fainting, chest pains, or leg swelling.

In April, 1996, the Food and Drug Administration (FDA) cleared the approval of dexfenfluramine, now known by its commercial name of Redux. An advisory panel to the FDA had previously concluded that Redux's benefits to obese persons —diminished risks for cardiovascular disease, diabetes, and some forms of cancer—outweighed any potential risks of the medication.

In its most basic terms, what this approval means is that we are seeing further validation of my basic premise that there is a specific biology to weight gain and that biological solutions are the answer. Clearly Redux holds great promise, but like most medications, it's not free of risk. You may be aware of the recent controversy surrounding the safety and efficacy of Redux. While there is a small risk of possible PPH, the enormous health benefit of losing weight usually outweighs it. I have already introduced Redux in my practice and have gained some experience with it. One of its possible advantages is that it may be less sedating, so I have switched selected fen-phen patients to a Redux/phentermine combination. In any case, your physician should carefully evaluate your risk/ benefit profile and discuss it with you.

The introduction of this new medication to the physician's armamentarium doesn't mean that Redux will automatically replace the use of fenfluramine. Tolerance of various drugs differs. Just as every heart patient doesn't have a positive response to diuretics or to calcium blockers, we can't expect every obesity patient to be successful on Redux. Some people will continue to do better on the old drugs, which is why I believe there will always be a place for fenfluramine and phentermine in the treatment of obesity.

Xenical

Xenical, less commonly known as tetrahydrolipistatin, is a drug not as far along as dexfenfluramine in the FDA-approval process. It is currently being tested in the United States and Europe, with 4,000 patients taking part in two-year trials.

Xenical differs from dexfenfluramine, fenfluramine, and phentermine in that it doesn't act on the brain's neurotransmitters. Instead, it helps to block the body's absorption of fat from foods.

Xenical blocks the activity of three lipases—the intestinal enzymes that break dietary fat down into absorbable components of monoglycerides and fatty acids. When taken three times a day, the drug prevents the absorption of about one-third of the fat eaten daily. This translates into a loss of 225 to 270 fat calories. In one study, subjects lost an average of 11 pounds in three months while taking the drug and following a moderate eating regimen, which was almost twice the amount of weight lost by the control group.

The drug's future depends not only on studies of its efficacy but also on the public's reaction to its rather unpleasant side effects. Since Xenical blocks fat absorption, stools tend to be greasy, bulky, and noxious. There may also be some accompanying diarrhea and flatulence. If these problems can be accepted, however, Xenical may well prove to be a suitable addition to the growing arsenal of anti-obesity medications.

Engineered Metabolic Changes

The *ob* gene is not the only discovery that opens up a role for genetic engineering in weight control. Another possibility concerns biotechnological alteration of metabolism. But to understand this option, we must first understand the function of so-called brown fat in the body.

Ninety-nine percent of body fat is composed of "white fat," the fat you see between your fingers, for example, if you squeeze your thigh or abdomen. The remaining one percent, "brown fat," is found in small amounts in your back and vital organs.

Brown fat cells look brown because they are packed with dark-colored mitochondria, the tiny organs that produce energy for the cell. Unlike white fat, which is virtually inert, researchers believe that the small deposits of brown fat burn like miniature furnaces, converting a few hundred calories taken in each day into energy. Because of its metabolic role, brown fat may hold one of the keys to weight loss. Scientists are currently looking for ways to stimulate brown fat activity even further to increase metabolism.

As with the *ob* gene, only research will tell whether this type of genetic engineering can be accomplished. LipoCyte, Inc., a biotechnology company in Lakewood, New Jersey, has a patent pending on a method that, when completely developed, would work like this: Tissue is removed from the patient's body with a syringe, sent to a laboratory where it is genetically engineered to raise metabolic rate, and then implanted back into the patient. The most usual site for implantation would be the back, but several locations might be used at once, depending on the amount of weight to be lost.

Once ideal weight is reached, a "suicide gene" could be implanted to wipe out the engineered heat cells. Then, for long-term weight maintenance, the heat cells would be replaced with slower-burning cells.

Company officials hope to begin FDA-approved clinical trials in two to four years. If successful, this new technology should be available to all physicians within ten years.

A Stomach-to-Brain Connection

While researchers are exploring the brown fat link to weight loss, researchers at Purdue University in Indiana are looking in another direction. They have found that the nerves in the digestive tract play a major role in controlling what we eat.

"It used to be thought that the brain got little or no feedback from the stomach, but this is not the case at all," says Terry L. Powley, Ph.D., professor of psychological sciences and director of the research. "There is a massive nerve network in the gastrointestinal tract that sends a lot of messages to the brain all the time. Stomach nerves assess every morsel that enters the body."

Powley's work, which was performed on rats, found that nerve endings monitor food from the time it touches the tongue until it completes its passage through the intestines. Using new technology that tracks neural sensors, Powley discovered that the vagus nerve, which runs from the central nervous system to the stomach, has a dense array of branches reaching into the stomach and intestines.

Given their complexity, number, and diversity, Powley describes these nerves as "major players" in the obesity equation. If a person is overweight, it may be because the neural network is inactive and not sending the brain correct information. Or, the nerves may be working, but not at an appropriate level.

Powley believes that if ways could be found to "harness the nerves, optimize their output, and take advantage of them, it would prove to be invaluable." He speculates that in the future medications may be developed or nutrients discovered that can harness the nerve feedback circuit for weight-control purposes.

The Future Is Here

As hard as it is to believe, what reads like science fiction is actually the future of not just obesity research and treatment but all of medicine. We are coming closer to a time when illness may be treated on an unprecedented genetic and biological level. Rather than treating symptoms and controlling the spread of disease, we will be increasingly able to trace and treat the biological cause of illnesses such as obesity.

After witnessing the incredible results of medical progress in the past twenty years, and seeing the tangible results of treatment with fenfluramine and phentermine in my practice on a daily basis, I look forward with excitement to the realization of even more effective pharmacological treatments for obesity. If obesity can be treated successfully in these ways, it is bound to produce a healthier population with fewer incidences of heart disease, stroke, diabetes, crippling arthritis, and certain forms of cancer.

I feel that I have given you the tools to begin to treat your own weight problem. My three-pronged approach to obesity—

combining sensible eating, regular exercise, and medications —will assuredly lead you to good health.

Now, why don't you begin living the rest of your life as a liberated person? Leave behind the exclusionary diet mentality that dominated a good part of your life. Get off that psychologically damaging roller coaster and take action.

Change always requires plenty of courage, and the first step you need to take right now is to acknowledge that you have a chronic medical condition called obesity, which must be treated and managed. Find a physician who can treat your condition properly. Don't ever let anyone badger or belittle you about your weight again.

In losing weight and keeping it off, my hope is that you will rediscover the joy that comes from moving. I want you to be awakened to healthful eating and improved nutrition. In doing so, you will be invigorated by increased self-esteem and will finally become the "normal" person you have always dreamed of being.

Be well, my friends!

CHAPTER TWELVE

Questions Patients Often Ask

Q. *Who is a good candidate for the drugs?*
A. There are a number of factors. Physically, you should be 20 percent over your ideal body weight. You also have to recognize that obesity is a major health risk that needs to be corrected. A study in the *New England Journal of Medicine,* for example, concluded that women who weighed 30 percent more than they should were three times more likely to die of heart disease than women of normal weight. If you know that your weight could cause you serious trouble, you're likely to be motivated to succeed on the medications.

You also have to be willing to take responsibility for your own health and well-being. This means eating a healthful diet, exercising regularly, and being prepared to use the medications over the long term. Psychologically, a good candidate understands that he or she will never be "cured," but may always have to rely on the drugs for assistance, as needed.

Q. *Who is a poor candidate for the medications?*
A. People who feel uncomfortable taking medications of any sort, whether for physiological or psychological reasons, will not feel comfortable on fenfluramine and phentermine. Included in this group are patients who can't put up with the discomfort of any sort of side effect—dry mouth, for example —even though side effects generally clear up in a reasonable amount of time. Similarly, individuals who are not committed to a complete program of weight reduction, including sensible eating and regular exercise, will not do as well as others on the drugs. Ultimately, I find, these patients drop the program or fail to keep their weight off.

Q. *How do I know when I am ready to take the medications?*
A. If you weigh more than 20 percent above your ideal weight, carry an excessive amount of body fat, and have been unable to maintain weight loss with traditional methods, you would be a likely candidate. Remember, though, that while phentermine and fenfluramine will help you to lose weight, taking the medications does not override your responsibility to exercise regularly and eat properly.

Q. *How do I get started with the medications?*
A. Consult with your family physician. If your doctor does not know about the drugs, suggest that he or she read the materials at the end of this book, or you can ask to be referred to a

colleague who is more familiar with the medications. You should not have to see a specialist in obesity to be put on a weight-loss program. Just as primary-care physicians treat such chronic ailments as asthma, diabetes, or hypertension, they should also be able to treat obesity and to prescribe the medications. Unfortunately, we're not quite there yet, but as more doctors and their patients realize the effectiveness of the medications, perceptions and medical treatment will start to change.

Q. *How fast will I lose weight after I start taking phentermine and fenfluramine?*
A. It depends on a number of factors. Men lose weight faster than women because they have more metabolically active tissue. If you restrict your caloric input and exercise regularly, you'll lose weight faster than someone who does neither of these things. If you are incapable of anything more vigorous than moderate walking to begin with, your loss will be slower than someone who can start off by bicycling twenty to thirty minutes a day.

Because people are so varied, you shouldn't be concerned with how much weight you'll lose or how fast you'll lose it. I can assure you, however, that weight loss will occur if you are able to tolerate the medications for four to twelve weeks. Ninety percent of my patients lose weight while taking the medications as prescribed.

Q. *Is either of the two drugs addictive?*
A. There is no research to suggest that either phentermine or fenfluramine is addictive. These drugs affect the brain's

neurotransmitters, working along more direct pathways than amphetamines, those highly addictive diet pills popular in the 1950s. Unfortunately, amphetamines, or "speed," have tainted the reputation of all subsequent obesity medications, making physicians and patients think the newer drugs are "speed," leaving them wary of using any drugs in obesity treatment.

Q. *At what time of day should I take the medications?*
A. Some physicians prescribe both drugs to be taken in the morning. However, I have suggested that patients who are on 15 mg of phentermine and 20 mg of fenfluramine take the phentermine before 11 A.M. to avoid any sleep problems and the fenfluramine at 5 P.M. For patients on higher doses of fenfluramine, another pill is taken each day before noon.

Q. *Why do I need to take both drugs?*
A. When used in combination, the drugs are far more effective than when using one drug alone. Phentermine is a mild stimulant; fenfluramine is a mild depressant. In tandem, they counteract each other's side effects. But if a patient cannot tolerate one of the medications, I do not hesitate to prescribe only the other. Often, these drugs can be used quite effectively by themselves.

Q. *What are the most usual side effects I can expect?*
A. The drugs—like many other medications—may cause dry mouth in some patients, but most people don't find this to be too uncomfortable. Other possible side effects are diarrhea, nausea, and mild stimulation, but the latter is often not un-

pleasant. Some people experience headache when the drugs are initiated. Most side effects clear up by the second week or so. It's important, however, to discuss any side effects you develop with your physician.

Q. *Are there any unusual side effects I should know about?*
A. It has been reported by some patients that the use of fenfluramine can lead to some minor memory loss. If this happens to you, you need to stop taking the medications. From all accounts, the loss is reversible once the drugs are discontinued.

Q. *When I take the medication, are there any dietary restrictions?*
A. No, but your goal should be to adopt better eating habits so that you improve your health and maintain weight loss with greater ease. I don't want my patients to feel deprived, however, so I don't recommend eliminating any foods. But I do suggest that high-fat foods should represent no more than 30 percent of your daily caloric intake and alcoholic beverages should be eliminated or at least limited.

Q. *Are there any conditions that would make it inadvisable for me to take either or both the medications?*
A. Yes. If you are prone to cardiac arrhythmias, where any change in heart rate would have negative effects, I would be reluctant to prescribe phentermine. I might recommend a low dose of fenfluramine, but you would have to be followed up regularly and seen every week to ten days.

If you have arthritis or lupus, take cortisone on a regular basis, and have gained weight because of the cortisone, I wouldn't put you on the anti-obesity medications. Unfortunately, the drugs have no effect in reducing weight caused by regular cortisone use.

Alcoholism makes use of the medications problematic, since the sedative effects of alcohol and fenfluramine in combination can have poor results. In any case, I would treat the alcoholism first and would not recommend either drug until the drinking was under control.

Q. *The medications reduce my appetite, but I try to reduce it further by not eating for a day or two. Is this a bad idea?*
A. Yes. It's not healthy to fast or starve yourself in an effort to lose weight because this weight loss—which is essentially from water—can't be maintained and you will eventually overeat in order to compensate. Fasting typically causes fatigue by reducing energy sources and changing electrolyte balances. Lack of food can also lead to low blood pressure, heart rhythm disturbances, and anemia. The bottom line: You shouldn't have to endanger yourself to lose weight.

Q. *Can I have a few alcoholic drinks a day when taking the medications?*
A. Because of the health dangers associated with alcoholism, I don't recommend excessive alcohol consumption for anyone. However, I have found that patients who drink moderately while on the drugs experience no untoward side effects. It's important to remember, though, that moderate consumption means no more than the equivalent of one ounce of pure alcohol per day. This is the amount found in two 12-ounce beers, two 5-ounce glasses of wine, or 1.5 ounces of spirits. Remember, too, that alcoholic beverages can add many calories to your diet without supplying nutrients.

Q. *How often do I need to see the doctor when I am on the drugs?*
A. It depends on the method your physician uses to evaluate, counsel, and monitor compliance. I give a patient a prescription for a one-month supply of the medications and set up an appointment for when the supply runs out. For those patients with special needs, I may see them weekly or every two weeks. That way, I can follow progress and adjust dosages, if necessary. It's important to stick to the schedule you establish with your physician.

Q. *Will my food urges always be under control when I'm taking the medications?*
A. Just as some days you may have been hungrier than others before you took the medications, you may have some days when appetite is greater, even when you're on the drugs. This is particularly likely to happen when you are under stress. If you experience a stress-related upsurge, don't increase the medications on your own. If you find that elevated appetite continues over a period of days, however, consult your physician. You may need to have your dosages increased.

Q. *I am 40 pounds overweight and take daily medication for high blood pressure. When I asked my family physician about taking diet medications, he said they would raise my blood pressure. Is this true? Can I take the drugs?*
A. I have found that phentermine may raise blood pressure slightly in some patients, which is why all medications must be monitored closely by a physician so that adjustments may be made as needed. I have not observed this with fenfluramine, nor is there any data to suggest it. The more important point, to my mind, is that obesity raises blood pressure more than

any other factor. Since you happen to be both obese and hypertensive, I believe you are a perfect candidate for the medications.

Q. *I've been taking the medications for two weeks and have lost only 4 pounds. What's wrong with me?*
A. Nothing. As long as the weight is coming off, and you are tolerating the medications, you'll continue to lose weight. Many people lose a great deal of weight quickly. For others, it can take as long as three months to see a significant impact. However, my advice is not to compare yourself with anyone else. Stick with the medication, be patient, continue to exercise regularly, and eat sensibly. Remember, too, you are not in a race to see how quickly you can lose weight. By adhering to this program, weight loss will occur—you can expect a loss of 15 percent of your body weight—and weight regain will not.

Q. *I weigh 100 pounds more than I should. I live in Tennessee. When I asked my physician if I was a good candidate for fenfluramine and phentermine, he told me that, unless I was in a clinical obesity study or had narcolepsy, he couldn't prescribe the medications for me. What can I do?*
A. In 1990—two years before Michael Weintraub's study was published proving the efficacy of using phentermine and fenfluramine for the long-term treatment of obesity—the state health department in Tennessee restricted the use of fenfluramine and phentermine. Health departments serve a very useful purpose and attempt to protect the public welfare. However, they are not always in the forefront when it comes to medical advances—even when scientific evidence is over-

whelmingly supportive. Sometimes, too, health departments make irrational decisions, often going against what leading medical experts agree upon.

I want to point out that each state health department has certain idiosyncrasies, some with reference to marriage licenses, some to HIV testing. With all of the accumulated studies, and the medical and public outcry for the use of medications in treating obesity, I am hopeful that the Tennessee health department will reevaluate its position and make an adjustment regarding the use of fenfluramine and phentermine. All patients are entitled to the best medical care and medical treatment should not be withheld on the basis of misconception, dogma, or in this case, guilt by wrongfully linking new medications with negative aspects of those that preceded them.

I suggest that you involve your physician and write to your state health department, your congressional representatives, and medical society, petitioning them to support a change in this ruling. In the meantime, seek medical attention in a nearby state from a physician who will treat you for your chronic medical condition. For referrals, contact The American Society of Bariatric Physicians, 5600 South Quebec, Suite 109A, Englewood, CO; tel. 303-779-4833.

Q. *A friend and I started taking the medications at the same time, but she's losing more weight than I am. Why?*
A. There are many variables involved in weight loss, such as how much muscle mass you have, how often you exercise, and how many calories you consume. That's why there is no one rate at which weight loss occurs. If you compare yourself with someone else, you're setting yourself up for emotional distress.

Since it's impossible to know why your friend is doing "better," why not forget about it?

Q. *I have a cholesterol reading of over 300. Will the medications help lower it?*
A. The medications won't lower your cholesterol directly, but by helping you lose weight, they may well bring about a reduction in cholesterol. This happens to the majority of people who are overweight and have high cholesterol, though there is no guarantee that the reduction will get you down to the recommended level of less than 200. Cholesterol is found only in food. To ensure that you have the best chance of achieving the goal of lowered cholesterol, eliminate egg yolks and limit consumption of meat and poultry to 3 ounces daily.

Q. *I recently lost 96 pounds and reached my goal weight by following a low-fat, low-calorie diet combined with regular exercise. In the two months since stopping the diet, I have put 12 pounds back on even though I continue to work out. I've been through this cycle before so many times, but I don't want to go on another diet. Am I a good candidate for the medications?*
A. Dieting, as you certainly know, is nothing but forced deprivation, but the moment you stop depriving yourself—as you did—the pounds start to accumulate. Reaching your goal weight is half of the struggle, but keeping the weight off is the most difficult part. You sound like a very good candidate for the medications. Since you have already lost most of your excess weight, your aim now is to keep the weight from coming back—and this is where the combination of phentermine and fenfluramine has proven to be so helpful. Combined with regular exercise and nutritious food choices, the medications

should help you lose the extra pounds and maintain your weight.

Q. *I am 75 pounds overweight and recently had a heart attack. Will I be able to take the medications?*
A. Yes, once your medical condition has been stabilized and you do not have uncontrolled hypertension or unstable cardiac arrhythmia (erratic heartbeats). A medically stabilized cardiac patient can be an excellent candidate for the drugs.

If you have a stable cardiac condition, then following consultation with your cardiologist, I would prescribe fenfluramine and phentermine.

Q. *I lost more than 160 pounds with the medications. Now I have sagging skin on my abdomen, arms, and thighs. My breasts sag, too. What do you recommend?*
A. When you have a lot of body fat, your skin stretches to accommodate it. When you lose the fat, your skin shrinks only somewhat, and a cosmetic condition like the one you describe develops. This is something that can't be cured by exercise or medication. There are two possible solutions. The first is to seek camouflage and comfort through clothing. Lycra undergarments, for example, will gently compress the flesh on your legs and abdomen, giving you a more pleasing profile. A push-up bra will lift sagging breasts, while long-sleeved blouses can conceal your arms.

The second option is plastic surgery. According to Manhattan plastic surgeon Barry Zide, this is a formidable process. But I have seen stunning results he has achieved with some of my patients. In some cases, such surgery is covered by medical insurance. If expense is a factor, limit the surgery to the skin problem you find most vexing. For referrals to board-certified plastic surgeons in your area, contact the American Society of Plastic and Reconstructive Surgeons (444 East Algonquin Road, Suite 110, Arlington Heights, IL 60005; tel. 708-228-9274).

Q. *I've been on the medications for two years and have reached my goal weight. My physician says it's time to stop the drugs, but I'm afraid of getting fat again. Will I?*

A. Your fear is somewhat justified in that weight tends to come back after the medications have been stopped. But if you follow a system of eating and exercise, you and your physician can taper off the drugs slowly when you reach your goal weight and see what happens.

Some people don't regain the weight at all. If my patients do put on 10 pounds or so, I "pulse" them—put them back on the medications for a time—until the weight is lost again. I tell them to regard the drugs as a safety net that's there for them, so fears of getting fat again need not be realized.

There is plenty of precedent for pulsing. When a depressed patient becomes stabilized, for example, I begin to reduce or stop the antidepressant medication. If the depression returns, I start the medication again until the depression lifts. In all cases involving chronic illness—and obesity is such an illness —it's better to return to the medication sooner rather than later.

Q. *I suffer from depression and I'm currently taking the antidepressant drug Paxil. Can I take phentermine and fenfluramine as well?*

A. I am not aware of any adverse drug interactions with Paxil, and I have no problem prescribing anti-obesity drugs for patients on that drug and, also, Prozac and Zoloft. However, the dosage of phentermine and fenfluramine may have to be adjusted for patients using antidepressant medications. I will not prescribe phentermine and fenfluramine to a patient being treated for depression with a monamine-oxidase inhibitor (MAOI) such as Nardil. The interaction of these drugs with other medications and certain foods creates the risk of stroke. You need to discuss your desire to take the anti-obesity drugs with the physician who prescribed your antidepressant.

Q. *I've just begun hormone replacement therapy after a hysterectomy, and I'm upset to find that I've put on 50 pounds. Can I take fenfluramine and phentermine along with the hormones?*
A. Yes. There is no adverse reaction between the drugs and the hormones. But be aware that the hormones aren't necessarily directly associated with weight gain. It's not uncommon to become depressed following surgery, decrease your activity level, and gain weight. Phentermine and fenfluramine, when used in conjunction with exercise and a healthy system of eating, can help you lose those unwanted pounds.

Q. *I find that many times I am not hungry when my family gets together to eat dinner. Should I force myself to eat with them?*
A. I always encourage families to eat at least one meal a day together so that they have a chance to bond, talk, and exchange ideas. If you're concerned about not being hungry at dinnertime, make sure to eat an early lunch and avoid having a late afternoon snack.

Q. *I am a diabetic who takes insulin. Can I take the medications?*
A. Diabetes does not preclude the use of the anti-obesity drugs, whether or not the person is on insulin. Weight reduction, combined with regular exercise and sound nutrition, can help all people with diabetes to manage their condition.

Q. *I am sixty-five years old and my body fat percentage is 46. Are the anti-obesity drugs effective for someone my age?*

A. Age is not a factor. As long as you are in good health and have no contraindications, such as uncontrolled hypertension or unstable cardiac arrhythmia, you are a good candidate for the drugs. And, of course, at any age, weight loss improves health and quality of life.

Q. *I'm planning to get pregnant sometime soon. Can I take the medications while I'm pregnant?*

A. No. As a safety precaution you should not take them if you are contemplating pregnancy in the next six months. Women should not take the medications while breast-feeding, either.

Q. *I will be having elective surgery soon. Can I continue the medications while I'm in the hospital?*

A. As a safety precaution, you should stop taking the medications a week before the surgery. Consult with your physician about when is the best time for you to resume your anti-obesity drugs. Since you will be using the drugs long term, being without them for a week or two won't have any lasting impact on your weight-loss efforts.

Q. *I have always had a tendency to gain weight but have managed to keep it in check with exercise and being careful about what I eat. Since I have been caring for my husband, who has Alzheimer's disease, I have put on 60 pounds in the past fifteen months. What can I do?*

A. Stress does play a role in weight gain and it is very predictable when people will gain weight. Since you do have a tendency to put on unwanted pounds, new psychological stresses in your life—either positive or negative—will directly impact on your weight. It's a biologic reality. Whenever people have changes in their life, such as a spouse's illness, starting a new job, going through financial reversals, suffering the death of a loved one, or going back to school for an advanced degree, I have found that those who are normally thin may gain weight and those who are heavy to begin with will become heavier.

If you are aware that you are affected by life's stresses and put on weight because of them, make sure that you keep up with your exercise routine and follow with your regular system of eating. If you are not taking the anti-obesity medications, this is a time when you should consider taking them. If you do take phentermine and fenfluramine, your physician may need to increase your dose or make some adjustment in your medication schedule.

Q. *I hate to exercise. Why should I have to if the medications will take off the weight?*
A. Exercise speeds up weight loss by building muscle and raising your metabolic rate, and it lowers cardiovascular risks. An added benefit: Regular exercise makes you feel better in body and spirit.

Q. *I weigh almost 50 pounds more than I should and have never exercised. What particular type of exercise do you recommend?*
A. You need to initiate exercise with great caution. First, consult your physician. You may need a complete physical as well as an exercise stress test, an important diagnostic test that is designed to uncover any cardiac abnormalities. Once you have a clean bill of health, your physician can design an appropriate exercise program for you, or you can join a fitness club that

has physiologists on staff, or you might even consider a personal trainer.

For a patient at the lowest level of fitness, I recommend slow walking, which can burn as many as 80 calories per mile. I also recommend a cross-country ski machine like the NordicTrack, an excellent exercise device that puts virtually no stress on your joints as you slide back and forth to fitness. As you start losing weight and become stronger, exercise intensity level can be raised and other activities introduced. The important point to remember is that moderation is the way to proceed.

Q. *I don't want to have large muscles. What's so great about weight training for women?*

A. Weight training helps you stay healthy because it builds muscles. The more muscle you have, the more quickly you burn calories. Also, as an added bonus, the more muscle you have, the more calories you will burn in the course of your everyday activities—even while you are sleeping. Researchers from the University of Florida have calculated that for every new ounce of muscle you build through exercise you will burn 25 percent more calories than any fat tissue it replaces.

A moderate training program creates a firmer, thinner physique, not oversized muscles. Body-builder muscles come from using heavy weights, performing fewer repetitions, and spending more time hoisting weights. Though women and men generally make the same strength gains, men have more muscle to show for it because of their high levels of testosterone, one of the primary hormones responsible for gains in muscle tissue. Before beginning a weight-training program, be sure to learn the proper lifting techniques from a certified trainer or some other experienced person.

Q. *I'm going on a cruise soon and I'm afraid I'll be tempted by the buffet meals. What can I do?*

A. Accept the fact that there's a natural tendency to overeat while on vacation. One thing you can do is watch the salt content of the new foods you encounter, since extra salt can cause water retention and weight gain. Generally, though, I tell my patients to relax, have a good time, and count on the pills to suppress appetite. Even if you overeat a bit, don't regard a few pounds gained as a tragedy. They can be lost on your return. It's a good idea, though, to exercise as much as possible on shipboard. If you can at least maintain your weight, that's a big plus.

Q. *How do I deal with Thanksgiving and other holidays?*

A. Enjoy your Thanksgiving meal. Remember that the pills will make you less hungry, so you can eat less, but still manage to sample just about everything. Remember, too, that people gain weight from a series of high-fat, high-calorie meals, not just one or two. Don't worry about your willpower. In fact, just don't worry, and have fun.

Q. *Why do I need to take prescription anti-obesity drugs when there are drugs available over the counter that can curb appetite?*

A. Unfortunately, most over-the-counter drugs contain phenylpropanolamine (PPA), a drug with similar chemical structure to that of amphetamine, or speed. PPA—introduced in 1979, and an ingredient of such popular diet pills as Acutrim and Dexatrim—can trigger alarming rises in blood pressure, which may result in stroke or death. The FDA is currently studying PPA. If a documented risk of stroke is found, all products containing PPA will probably be made available by prescription only. Fenfluramine and phentermine are both FDA-approved medications with few side effects and no known risk of stroke.

Q. *My insurance carrier will not pay for medications or office visits. When are these companies going to realize that obesity is a disease, and a chronic one at that?*

A. If obesity as a medical diagnosis is not covered under your plan, it is quite possible that an alternative diagnosis that you have, such as hypertension, diabetes, sleep apnea disorder, degenerative arthritis, or hiatal hernia, is covered by your policy. The good news is that more and more companies are reimbursing the primary diagnosis of obesity. However, since you are not covered under your current policy, have your physician write a letter on your behalf justifying your treatment to the medical director of your insurance company. Also, include the special tear-out section for physicians at the end of the book.

If possible, review other available plan options. Beyond that, I fear that the attitude of some insurance carriers is consistent with the overall discrimination against overweight people in this country. The American Heart Association has recognized obesity as being one of the primary risk factors for heart disease. So treatment for obesity is about more than personal appearance. It's about survival. By seeking medical treatment for obesity from your physician, you are certainly taking a positive step. As the scientific community moves toward accepting the notion of obesity as a chronic disease, the insurance companies will follow suit. In the near future, I hope that writing "obesity" on an insurance form will be sufficient to process your claim.

Q. *I am currently more than 60 pounds overweight. Will I be at risk of being turned down for life insurance because I am being treated with a medication for obesity?*

A. It's being overweight that makes you a health risk and, consequently, less desirable to an insurance company. The medications correct the problem, decrease your risk, and make you, to my way of thinking, more insurable.

Q. *I forgot to take my medications when I went away for a long weekend. I'm afraid I may have gained a lot of weight. Should I increase my dosage to make up for the lost days?*

A. When you go off your medications, you may start to feel some mild hunger. Also, if you had been on a high dose of fenfluramine, you may start to feel mild depression. In general, however, it is not a problem if you forget to take your medications. Simply restart your medications at the standard dosage you had been on.

As for your fears of instant weight gain after being off the drugs for four days: Gaining weight is a *gradual* process, so allay your fears about putting on a lot of weight in a short period of time.

Q. *I am fifty-eight years old, 5' 1", and weigh 193 pounds. I would like to take the medications. I have glaucoma and already take medication for this condition. Will the addition of the obesity drugs pose any problems for me?*

A. At your height, you probably need to lose 40 or more pounds. Phentermine and fenfluramine would certainly help you lose the weight when combined with regular exercise and sensible eating. However, since you are already taking medication for glaucoma, an eye disease that is one of the leading causes of blindness in this country, it is important that you mention to your ophthalmologist your desire to start with phentermine and fenfluramine. Have your primary-care physician speak with your ophthalmologist to get final approval.

Q. *I have heard of reports linking fenfluramine and dexfenfluramine with a serious illness called primary pulmonary hypertension. What are the risks for me if I take the medications?*

A. Infinitesimal. This does not negate the fact that any medication can pose a risk, however, which is why fenfluramine, dexfenfluramine, and phentermine should be used only by the appropriate patients. Primary pulmonary hypertension (PPH) is an extremely rare lung disorder with no known cause. At one time experts thought the disease occurred among young and middle-aged female subjects almost exclusively. Now it's known that males and females in all age ranges, from very young children to elderly people, can get PPH. Although millions of people have used fenfluramine-based medications, fewer than 50 case reports of PPH with the use of these drugs have been published. All of the patients were female. When dosages were specified, they were extremely high, with many taking 120 mg of fenfluramine a day. The risk of these medications should be compared to the extremely high mortality and sickness rates directly caused by obesity. Ultimately, you and your doctor need to determine what constitutes an acceptable risk for you.

Dexfenfluramine presents a different risk profile. Based on recent data from the International Primary Pulmonary Hypertension Study, investigators say the risk of developing PPH for patients using Redux (dexfenfluramine) is currently estimated to be between 23 and 46 cases per million patients per year.

Resources

Exercise Motivation

Although we all make promises to ourselves about getting in shape, most of us never make it past the "good intentions" stage. Here are some tips on how to make your resolutions more productive.

Commit to exercising regularly. You'll feel better knowing that the more consistently you exercise, the more you reduce the risk of dying from a serious disease.

Add just a bit more activity at first. Refrain from impulsively joining a health club or purchasing expensive equipment. Instead, begin by putting more physical activity into your daily routine by walking up the stairs instead of taking an elevator, for example, or parking your car at the far end of the supermarket parking lot so that you'll have to walk a little extra distance. Try to set aside at least some time each day to raise your activity level. Once you have increased activity over a two-to four-week span, you're ready to begin an organized exercise program.

Build the program gradually. After you decide on an exercise, begin by doing it a maximum of two days a week. It's a mistake to try to do too much, too soon. If you can keep your initial efforts at reasonable intensity, you have a better chance of succeeding as you expand the amount of time spent on exercise.

Take convenience into account. If you're planning to join a health club, make sure it's close enough to your home or workplace. If you want to start walking or running, be certain you're near a park, track, or some other suitable space.

Be kind to yourself. Don't get down on yourself if you miss your routine, and don't try to catch up by doubling up on the amount of exercise you usually do. Moderation and self-support are the keys to maintaining your enthusiasm.

Getting Started

Based on the experiences of my patients, here are some effective ways to begin:

- Take up the challenge of an activity you have never done before or one you haven't done recently. Good possibilities include bicycle riding, aerobic dance, water aerobics, scuba diving, or just plain walking.

- Make an appointment with a friend to do something active together every week.
- Take a walk with your spouse before dinner; take your children on walks around the neighborhood; join a walking group in your area.
- Go on a weekend hiking and camping trip.
- If possible, walk or ride your bicycle to do errands or to get to work.
- Play a tape of your favorite music and start dancing. If enthusiasm builds, sign up for dance lessons.
- Take your dog for a walk twice a day. If you don't have a dog, consider buying or adopting one.
- Make it a rule not to eat your lunch until you've gone for a walk or finished your workout.
- Sign up for a bicycle trip.
- Plan to take part in some type of appropriate athletic event, such as a walk for hunger or another good cause.
- Buy a new or used stationary bike, a treadmill, or a ski machine and place it near the television set. That way, you can do your thirty minutes or more of exercise a day and watch television at the same time.

Workout Structure

After getting clearance from your physician to begin, make sure that your workouts contain the following phases:

Warm-up phase (5 to 10 minutes): Gradually increase the workload of your heart and lungs and raise your body temperature by performing your activity at an easy pace. If you are walking, for example, start slowly and gradually pick up speed. Stretch the muscles you will be using—leg muscles in the case of walking—once they have become warm.

Exercise phase (20 to 60 minutes): During this phase, you do the activity at your full pace. If you've been completely sedentary, begin with exercise sessions of five to ten minutes two to three times a week. As you get stronger, increase your time to fifteen to thirty minutes or longer, and the number of sessions to four times a week.

Cool-down phase (10 to 15 minutes): Exercise can cause your heart and lungs to pump with twice their normal effort. Coming to a complete stop may make you dizzy or put a strain on your heart. Ease into three to five minutes of low-intensity aerobic exercise—walking slowly, for example—followed by a few minutes of stretching.

If you experience any of the following symptoms during or after exercise, contact your physician: dizziness, heavy sweating, rapid or irregular heartbeats, unusual shortness of breath, or increased chest, jaw, back, or arm pain.

Walking Basics

According to polls, walking is the most popular physical activity in the United States. Walking is excellent for overweight people because it is so gentle on the joints.

Start by mapping out a route for yourself. If you're planning to walk a mile, for example, drive your car a distance of one mile and return to your starting point. The same day, or the next, walk that measured mile and check your watch. To determine your walking speed, divide the number of minutes it took you to walk the mile into 60. If you walked the mile in 15 minutes, for example, your walking speed is 4 miles per hour.

A good walking pace for a beginner is 3 miles per hour, which means you will walk a mile in 20 minutes. As you get stronger, you'll want to follow my "rule of four": Walk four times a week for an hour at 4 miles per hour.

If you find you're not losing weight as rapidly as you want to, walk more often, not faster. An hour of easy walking at 3 miles per hour will burn the same number of calories as a half-hour of more strenuous walking at 4.5 miles per hour.

There are many ways to make your walking more effective and pleasurable:

- Walk with your spouse or a friend at least some of the time.
- Vary the lengths of your walks, the routes, the times of day, and your partners.
- Maintain a regular, comfortable stride.
- Walk so that you push off with all your toes at the same time, roll forward on the outside of your foot, and land on the outside corner of your heel.
- Keep your back straight and your head level.
- Bend slightly at the hips, not at the waist.
- Swing your arms gently back and forth for balance and rhythm.

Health and Safety Precautions for Walking

- Make sure your shoes are comfortable and strong. They should offer support around the heel, flexibility in the sole, and plenty of room around your toes.

- In cold weather, layer your clothing to retain heat. If walking in the dark, wear light-colored clothing to make yourself visible to motorists.

- If you must wear headphones, make sure they are turned down low and not placed fully in your ears.

- In the city, walk in the middle of sidewalks, rather than close to the buildings or parked cars.

- Don't walk in deserted areas.

- Tell someone where you plan to walk and when you expect to return. Carry identification, and take along enough change for a phone call, just in case.

- If you develop any type of ache or pain, or unusual shortness of breath, stop and return home. If necessary, seek medical aid.

Water Exercise Basics

When you exercise in shoulder-deep water, you weigh only 10 percent of what you weigh on land. Since the buoyancy supports you and cushions your joints, you avoid the strain so common with land-based activities. Surprisingly gentle as water is, you get a good workout when you perform an activity against its resistance, which is fourteen to sixteen times greater than what you would experience on land.

Other than a bathing suit, you need little equipment. You may want to buy an inexpensive life vest to keep your head above water in deep-water exercise. For shallow water, an old pair of running shoes can prevent your feet from blistering. For added leg resistance, wear an old pair of sweat pants. After five minutes in the water, you'll feel as if you have 10 pounds of weight strapped to your legs.

The beauty of working in a pool is that any kind of movement is effective, including a water aerobics class. If you don't opt for such a class, try either or both of these workouts:

Shallow water walking/running. Walk or run from one side of the pool to the other, lifting your knees up and down. Keep your posture erect and move your arms vigorously from side to side.

One procedure is to keep going until you feel tired. Another is to go from one side of the pool to the other, rest for a minute, and then return to the starting side, repeating the routine five to ten times or until you are tired. Afterward, cool down for five to ten minutes by walking slowly, without lifting your knees up and down.

Deep-water running. Wear a life vest and stay as erect as you can while balancing yourself in the water. Lift your thigh, stretch out your leg, and stride forward. Then push your leg down and behind you, bending it as you try to kick yourself in the buttocks. Repeat with the other leg. Run tall with your hips always in line with your shoulders. Don't let your buttocks drift backward. Swing your arms slightly. Breathe naturally.

One approach is to run in place for five to twenty minutes. If this becomes boring, run up and down the length of the pool. After the workout, cool down for five minutes by running easily, slowly moving your arms and legs back and forth.

Stationary Bicycling Basics

Bicycling for twenty- to forty-five-minute sessions three times a week will strengthen your leg muscles, the largest muscles in your body. Especially important is the added strength cycling gives to the muscles, tendons, and ligaments surrounding the fragile knee joints. It also slims your calves, tightens your buttocks, and tones your thighs. Other benefits include a reduced resting heart rate, expansion of the blood-transport system, speeded-up fat metabolism, and strengthening of the lower back muscles. The support given to the upper body makes stationary bicycling an excellent aerobic conditioner for people whose back or joint disorders prevent them from participating in other forms of exercise.

It's important to make sure that your bicycle has a seat, also called a saddle, that's appropriate for you. If you're interested primarily in comfort, look for a well-cushioned seat or buy a gel-filled seat cushion to cover the saddle. Remember, though, that the wider the seat, the greater the tendency to restrict pedaling motion, chafe your thighs, and bounce slightly as you pedal. Also, the more cushioned the seat, the greater the tendency for your hips to roll, thus curtailing the power that should go into pedaling.

If you want to increase pedaling efficiency, look for a bike that can be fitted with a variety of saddle models. You may want to substitute a leather-covered, plastic saddle, like the type found on most road and mountain bikes, for a cushioned saddle.

Saddle Adjustment for Standard Stationary Bicycles

If your saddle is set too high, you'll hyperextend your knee, that is, straighten it more than 180 degrees. If the saddle is set too low, you can overstress the ligaments and tendons surrounding the knee joints. Follow these rules of thumb to fit your saddle properly:

- Make sure the saddle is perpendicular to the ground.
- When seated on the bike in your cycling shoes, place your heels on the pedals. You should be able to pedal backward with no discernible rocking motion in your hips.
- When you are pedaling, there should be a 15-degree bend in your knee at the bottom of the downstroke. Adjust your seat post accordingly.
- Wearing a good pair of form-fitting bicycling shorts with padding provides the most comfortable workout. Unlike cotton or nylon, these shorts will not bunch up in the crotch or chafe your inner thigh as you pedal. If you prefer unpadded shorts, choose a close-fitting pair with minimal seams.

Recumbent Bicycles

Recumbent bikes, about the height of a regular chair for most models, are lower to the floor than standard exercise bicycles. You sit in a partially supine position with your legs stretched out to the pedals in front, while your back is fully supported. Since these bikes are easy to get in and out of, they are a safer choice, particularly for exercisers with physical limitations.

Recumbents are excellent for people who are just starting a fitness regimen because, at the lowest setting, they are easier to pedal. Also, the large stable seat is more comfortable for those who have low back pain.

Wind Trainers

If you already have a road or mountain bike, an alternative to a stationary bike is to buy a wind trainer. These devices, also called "wind loaders" or "mag resistance trainers," are lightweight, aluminum stands that have either small fans or electromagnets. To use them indoors, you place the rear tire of your bike on the spindle of the trainer. Both fan and magnet models work on the same principle of simulating wind resistance when you pedal. The faster you pedal, the greater the resistance, and the feeling you get is the same as if you were outdoors.

Getting Started on the Stationary Bicycle

In your first few sessions, you may feel a burning sensation in your chest after a couple of minutes. This is nothing to worry about, and it will go away as your physical conditioning improves.

Also in the beginning, your mouth may feel as if it's filled with cotton, and your legs may feel leaden. These sensations will also disappear as you get into better shape.

Leg cramps, however, should not be ignored. If you experience them, get off the bike immediately, knead the cramped muscles, then walk around a bit and take a drink of water. Get back on the bike, reset the resistance to a lower level, and continue your workout.

In your first session, set the resistance at low, and concentrate on becoming acquainted with your bike. If you feel good after five minutes of pedaling, try pushing the resistance up a bit higher, pedal for forty to fifty turns, and then lower the resistance again. Repeat several times until you get a feel for the higher resistance and what it does to your legs and lungs. Remember that this is only a test to see what your bike and your body are capable of.

In the following sessions, work to build an aerobic base by pedaling at a steady, nonstop pace, and raising resistance gradually. It's safest to work at a level that's slightly below your maximum ability, so that you don't become exhausted or burned out. This type of pedaling is called LSD, an acronym for long steady distance, and it allows you to come to your next workout feeling refreshed and ready to ride again.

Here are some additional tips for cycling success:

- Don't become dehydrated. Take a drink of water every five minutes, even if you don't feel thirsty. Lack of water can cause your muscles to overheat and to cramp.

- Get a small fan and position it so that it cools your legs and upper body as you pedal.

- Make the time pass by listening to your favorite music, watching TV, or watching a video.

- Maintain your bike properly. Even a low-maintenance bike will need some lubrication to keep giving a smooth ride. Check your owner's manual for recommendations.

Resistance Training Basics

There are several ways to learn resistance training exercises, also called weight lifting. If you want to teach yourself from a book, I recommend *Getting Stronger* by Bill Pearl (Shelter Publications), which I consider the "bible" for trainers of all ability levels.

You can also ask a friend who is skilled at weight lifting or a professional instructor to teach you how to perform the exercises. Most health clubs and fitness centers now provide such instructors. The person should show you how to use each piece of equipment properly, how to decide on how much weight to use, and how to keep your routines interesting. It's easy for a beginner to pick up bad habits, and a good instructor will correct them early on.

A Resistance Training Workout

Resistance workouts should be scheduled every other day at most, so that you have a full day's rest in between. A typical workout includes a five- to ten-minute warm-up (skipping rope or running in place), followed by a routine of approximately twelve exercises, half for the lower body and half for the upper body.

Your goal is to tax your muscles. Start with light weights that you can lift comfortably ten to fifteen times. These repetitions of a specific exercise form a set. Perform two to three sets of each exercise with a one- to two-minute rest period in between. Remember that at the beginning your muscles may be sore. This is nothing to worry about. It's simply a sign that your muscles are expanding.

As you become stronger, increase the weight slightly. If you have difficulty performing the movements, return to the lower weight for a while. Over time, add exercises to the routine that use your own body weight, such as push-ups and crunches. For an unbeatable weight-loss program, combine weight lifting with low-fat eating and some form of regular aerobic exercise, such as walking, bicycling, or water aerobics.

Tips for creating your own light weights: To make two one-pound weights, take a pair of old athletic socks, put three rolls of pennies in each, and knot the tops. Soup cans can also be used as weights. Homemade weights can be used for arm curls, overhead presses, and other standard motions.

Personal Trainers

A decade ago, most personal trainers were self-taught athletes who knew what worked for them and passed the knowledge along to clients. Today's trainers have the opportunity for education and certification, but even as the profession evolves, no state has legislated licensing requirements. Currently, anyone can put on a T-shirt and a pair of Lycra shorts and announce that he or she is a trainer.

If you are interested in pursuing the option of a personal trainer, one way is to work with a trainer at a reputable health club. Top clubs hire trainers with degrees in physical education and backgrounds in anatomy or kinesiology, the science of human movement. Clubs also look for experience in teaching a sport and certification from a professional organization, such as the National Strength and Conditioning Association. Many clubs also require trainers to earn continuing education credits every two years.

If you want a trainer who will come to your house, a local health club or sports medicine clinic may be willing to give you some names. Another way, since most trainers depend on word of mouth, is simply to ask around among your friends and associates.

You can also contact the following educational and certifying organizations:

American Council on Exercise
Box 910449
San Diego, CA 92191-0449
(800-234-9229)
Provides regional personal trainer referrals.

Certified Strength and Conditioning Agency
P.O. Box 83469
Lincoln, NE 68501-3469
(402-476-6669)
A branch of the National Strength and Conditioning Association, this group provides regional trainer referrals through state directors.

National Academy of Sports Medicine
2434 North Greenview Avenue
Chicago, IL 60614
(312-929-5101)
Provides certified fitness trainer referrals.

Many trainers are available for consultation via phone and fax machine. Michael Margulies, director of MedFit (212-249-8122), who works with many of my patients, offers this service.

Once you have the names of several trainers, learn as much as you can before choosing one. In a half-hour interview, ask the trainer to explain his or her workout methods and the reasoning behind them. Make sure the trainer has a background in exercise physiology, anatomy, injury prevention, and the monitoring of exercise intensity.

If you have a past injury or a medical condition, such as hypertension, diabetes, or asthma, ask how the trainer would customize a program for you. The trainer should also be willing to discuss workout plans with your physician and to apprise the doctor of your progress over time.

Good listening skills and an ability to communicate are critical. As with learning any sport, you need a teacher whose personality makes you feel comfortable. If you're a pretty easygoing type, for example, and you select a marine sergeant, you're not likely to achieve your workout goals.

The sex of the person also has to be taken into account. Some people feel more comfortable working with someone of the same sex, others with someone of the opposite sex. You need to know your own preferences or if sex matters at all.

Certification from a nationally recognized organization is highly desirable. It means that the individual, in addition to having training skills, is also certified in cardiopulmonary resuscitation (CPR) and first aid. If you must use a noncertified trainer, make sure that he or she has at least passed a CPR course. It's also important for the trainer to have liability insurance and to give you the names of references you can check out.

A good test is to hire a trainer who seems suitable for one or two sessions and ask yourself these questions: Am I getting along with this person? Am I learning? Do I feel motivated?

Enthusiasm is a prized skill in a trainer, and it's one that can't be measured by any certification test. The person you hire should be able to charm, cajole, and prod you to achieve your goals, while sustaining your level of motivation. If a trainer has all the enthusiasm of an IRS agent, the chances that you will adhere to the program are slim. But if you select someone whose attitude makes you feel like a million bucks, you could wind up looking that way, too. But remember, a trainer is an option, not a necessity.

Alternative Ways of Exercising

If you need a change of pace from your routine, or if you want to work out while traveling, you can use a video, work along with a television fitness show, or go to a health club. Here are some points to consider about each.

The Exercise Video

Choose the right video and you can have a private workout at home whenever you want one. However, a well-sculpted body on the box doesn't always mean a safe and effective workout inside. With so many tapes available, it can be difficult to separate the good from the useful or even potentially injurious.

It's a good idea to rent a video from your local store or library before you buy it. Watch the entire routine before you perform it, asking yourself these questions:

- Is this tape geared to someone on my level?
- Does the tape recommend that viewers consult their physicians before using it?

- Is the leader a recognized exercise expert?
- Has the tape been endorsed by a reputable sports medicine association?
- Are there appropriate warm-up and cool-down periods?
- Does the leader explain how easy or difficult various movements will be?
- Are alternatives offered to vigorous or challenging movements?
- Is there an explanation of how to monitor your pulse, and when to stop if you feel discomfort?
- Can I easily adapt this routine to my needs?

Whether a tape deals with stretching, kick-boxing, or stair climbing, you should be able to answer most of these questions in the affirmative. What you are looking for is a sensible routine, conducted by a qualified leader, with clear instructions to the viewer. Choose wisely when you rent or purchase, and you can come away with a substantial fitness routine.

The Television Show

If you're an early riser, turn on the television set, and get ready to move to the one-two beat of some of the best workout stars. These exercise gurus have many loyal followers, but is it really possible to get a safe workout in the glow of the cathode tube? Won't you push too hard and perhaps strain yourself?

There's little reason to worry. Many leading instructors have degrees in physical education and conduct classes when they're not in front of the cameras. On television, as in their classes, they explain how to perform an exercise, which body part it is working, and how to follow safety precautions.

The shows are also planned properly so that they progress from a warm-up period, to a 20-minute segment of aerobic exercises, to a brief cool-down period. Many programs vary their formats, sometimes offering flexibility, toning, and shaping exercises instead of aerobics after the warm-up.

The bottom line in evaluating a fitness show is whether it inspires you to exercise or just sit back and watch. To be effective, you need to work out with the show on a regular basis.

It can help to follow these tips:

- If you are just beginning an exercise program, check with your physician first. Be sure to describe the physical demands of the program.
- Be prepared to exercise before you turn on the set. Have an exercise mat in place. Wear your favorite sweats, a leotard, or shorts.
- Make a commitment to exercise with the program for several weeks before judging the results.
- If you know you'll have to miss an airing of the show, videotape it, and exercise later on.
- Don't rely solely on the program, even if it becomes your exercise foundation. For variety, walk, swim, or ride a bike several times a week.

The Health Club

Quality health clubs provide aerobics, step, and slideboard classes, resistance exercise equipment, and the facilities to perform such sports as swimming, racquetball, tennis, and basketball. Many clubs offer fitness assessment, physical therapy, nutritional counseling, and massage therapy. Some even have a social component, such as dinners, theme parties, and excursions to sporting events. Consider your own personal needs as you evaluate a club.

Before joining any club, inspect the facility for utilization level. Ideally, go at a time when the club is likely to be busy, such as lunch hour or before or after work. If the crowds are too large, you're likely to have to spend a lot of time waiting instead of exercising, and the staff may be too busy to provide individual instruction. Without attention, you can develop bad form, particularly in resistance training, and injuries may result.

Here are some other points to consider:

Location. Make sure the club is close enough to your home or office to reach it conveniently. If you have to travel too far, you'll soon have a laundry list of excuses for not exercising.

Size. Workout rooms and classrooms should be spacious enough to accommodate members comfortably without a sense of crowding. Try using a stationary bicycle or weight machine. If you feel that other machines are too close to yours, or that too many people are working out nearby, the facility is not spacious enough.

Instructors. Ask about the education and training required of instructors and the amount of personal attention they are prepared to give each member. What is the ratio of instructors to members? If possible, chat with some of the instructors before making a decision to join.

Program. Does the club have the activities you're interested in pursuing? If a club specializes in aerobic dance, for example, and lacks the stair-climber classes you want, it may not be the place for you.

Equipment. Look for a variety of up-to-date workout and weight-resistance machines. Each machine should have clear instructions for use. The equipment doesn't have to be brand new, but it does have to be well maintained. Grungy machines can put a damper on your motivation to exercise, and they can be dangerous, too.

Lockers. Are there enough lockers and are they large enough to hold your business attire without wrinkling it? If lockers are in short supply, find out if there are other safe places for storing your valuables.

Showers. There should be enough showers so that you won't have to stand on line to use them. Inspect for cleanliness, too. A messy shower room is a tip-off to a poorly run facility. Other things to consider: Are fresh towels available? And, if you think you'll want more than a shower, does the club have a steam room, sauna, or hot tubs?

Child care. If you plan to bring young children with you, you'll need a place that offers child care. Many top clubs provide a supervised playroom and planned activities. If the club you're considering is heavily utilized, make sure the children's room isn't overcrowded and that supervision is sufficient.

Guests. Is there a special fee for guests? Is there a limit to the number of visits one guest can make?

Health clubs can vary substantially in price, depending on the number of amenities offered. Usually, the costs include an initiation fee as well as yearly dues. Most clubs, however, have trial memberships at reduced or no cost. Look for these in the newspaper and in the mail. By taking advantage of a special offer, you can evaluate the club and decide whether you want to continue the membership.

Exercise on the Road

An extended business trip or vacation needn't put an end to your exercise program. A workout away from home can be stress-relieving and fun, if you plan ahead.

Before you book a hotel, ask about the facilities. Many good hotels have an exercise room with a complete array of equipment. Also find out if there's an indoor pool. At the very least, the hotel should be near a health club where you can work out or a park where you can walk or run. If the hotel doesn't have what you need, explain why you won't be staying there. When guests speak up, managers listen, and the next time you travel to the area, the hotel may be better equipped.

One of the advantages of being on the road is that you can be creative about your exercise. Come up with a workout that's a change of pace. If you walk or run at home, try a stationary bike or swimming laps. Arrange to participate in a couple of aerobics classes at a nearby health club. Another option, if you have a room with a VCR, is to rent an exercise video. Some hotels even provide such videos, along with simple equipment, such as bench steps.

Since business or even vacation schedules are likely to be hectic, make exercise appointments with yourself. If you usually exercise in the morning at home, but you've got early meetings on the road, pencil in a workout from 4 to 5 in the afternoon. There's even a business advantage here. By exercising later in the day, you'll go to dinner meetings or social events feeling refreshed.

The key to exercising on the road is to accept limitations. Leave the strenuous workouts for the familiar surroundings of home. Instead, work out at a moderately elevated heart rate, simply to main fitness. If you can do that, you'll relieve the stress of business travel, and you'll return home free from guilt about not having exercised.

The Smoker's Weight Dilemma

Smokers tend to be thinner than nonsmokers because something in tobacco, most likely nicotine, causes the body to handle fat in a different way. This process, called lipolysis, frees lipids, or fats, from fat-storing cells and spills them into the bloodstream. Some of these fats are burned by the higher metabolism smoking creates, while others are converted by the liver into triglycerides, which clog the arteries. Even as the increased metabolism keeps weight down, the triglycerides contribute to the high incidence of heart disease among smokers—a poor trade-off.

Still, many smokers fear they will eat more and gain weight if they quit. It is true that the average smoker gains 10 pounds within a year of quitting, and one in eight gains 30 pounds, but this is not necessarily due to increased eating. A study at the University of California at Berkeley found that people who stop smoking might actually eat less and still put on pounds.

If you're contemplating quitting, the sensible way to avoid weight gain is to increase exercise levels to compensate for the metabolic "advantages" of smoking. Let's assume that moderate smoking keeps off 200 calories a day. You should be able to burn off the same amount by walking 2 miles in forty-five minutes, and you don't need to risk your health to do it.

Vital Statistics

Bathroom scale weight should not be the only determinant of whether or not you have a weight problem. Leading researchers use the following methods to determine whether health is being compromised by body type and size. Use these handy guides to achieve a more accurate assessment of your own health profile.

Body Weight Distribution

Obesity has traditionally been defined as weighing 20 percent more than your ideal weight, as determined by the Metropolitan Life Insurance tables. However, researchers now believe that where the fat is located is more important than how much you weigh.

If most of your fat is on your hips and thighs, making you

pear-shaped, you are less at risk for health problems than if most of the fat is on your abdomen, making you apple-shaped. Abdominal fat is more dangerous because the fatty acid content of these fat cells goes directly to the liver before circulating to the muscles. It becomes more difficult for the liver to clear insulin from the bloodstream, blood glucose levels rise, and the pancreas produces more insulin. The increased insulin triggers the release of norepinephrine, a brain chemical that causes blood pressure to rise. If the cycle continues, your chances of developing adult-onset diabetes, hypertension, stroke, and other diseases increase dramatically.

Thus, body shape can be more important than weight when it comes to health. A thin apple-shaped person, for example, is at greater risk than an obese pear-shaped person. That's why it's important to know where you are carrying weight by determining your waist-to-hip ratio. A man's waist-to-hip ratio should be 0.85 and a woman's should be between 0.7 and 0.75.

To calculate, do the following:

- Using a cloth tape measure, have someone measure your waist at its narrowest point above the navel. Measure to the nearest quarter inch.
- Measure your hips at their widest point.
- Divide your waist measurement by your hip measurement, rounding out to the nearest tenth.

Example: Mary has a waist measurement of 35 and a hip measurement of 44. Her waist-to-hip ratio is 0.795, or 0.8. She divided 35 by 44 to arrive at this number. Mary's number is above the safe range for women.

Body Mass Index

The body mass index (BMI) measures the relationship of your weight to your height. You can use the index to determine whether your weight is low enough to protect you from obesity-related ailments.

To figure out your BMI, use a calculator for the math and follow these steps:

1. Weigh yourself without clothing and divide the pounds by 2.2.

2. Measure your height in stocking feet and divide the inches by 39.4. Multiply the number you get by itself.

3. Divide the results of step 1 by the results of step 2. The desirable BMI range for males is 21.9 to 22.4 and for females 21.3 to 22.1.

Body-Fat Percentage

It is body fat, not weight per se, that causes health problems and makes overweight people look large. By knowing the proportion of fat in your body, you can take steps to rid yourself of the excess.

Your physician may be able to gauge body-fat composition by using a computerized test, a near-infrared device, or skin-fold calipers. Many sports medicine clinics, health clubs, and registered dietitians also offer this service. It is possible to track your body fat in the privacy of your home with professional-quality, inexpensive skin-fold calipers. Accu-Measure, Inc. (P.O. Box 4040, Parker, CO 80134; tel. 800-866-2727) sells a quality product for approximately $20.

Be aware that the margin of error in most body-fat testing can be as high as 5 percent. Nevertheless, a ballpark figure is probably useful enough. A high reading can serve as a warning that you need to exercise more frequently and lower your intake of dietary fat.

Body-Fat Ranges

Males: Optimal: 10% to 15%
          Average: 18% to 23%
          Obese: 25% or more

Females: Optimal: 17% to 22%
          Average: 25% to 29%
          Obese: 35% or more

FOR YOUR PHYSICIAN
(Photocopy or cut out)

Dear Doctor:

We can all agree that obesity has had a negative impact on the health of our patients. It's certainly obvious that the available treatments have been ineffective and inadequate. If you are as frustrated as I had been in the management of obesity, then reading the following information will be useful to you.

The past ten years have resulted in exciting new information in the field of obesity. Studies by Rockefeller University researchers Sarah Leibowitz, Ph.D., on neuropeptides, Jeffrey Friedman Ph.D., on the *ob* gene, and Jules Hirsch, M.D., on setpoint theory are making it very clear that obesity is a chronic *medical* disease requiring *medical* solutions.

Telling patients to reduce caloric intake and increase exercise is not enough to overcome the genetic and metabolic propensity to obesity. For me, the most effective approach in treating my obese patients has been with the use of the anorectic drugs, fenfluramine and phentermine, used in combination, and in some instances, individually. The use of the drugs does not obviate the need for patients to follow appropriate nutrition guidelines, to exercise, and to modify behavior. The drugs do, however, provide relief from suffering, produce concrete results in real weight loss, and offer hope for management of this chronic disorder.

Drug therapy for obesity, as I am sure you are aware, has been discouraged because of the prior use of amphetamine-

237

based medications. Phentermine and fenfluramine, however, are not amphetamines. Contrary to what you may read in the PDR, these drugs can be used for more than twelve weeks; there is no current data to support a claim of addictiveness. Moreover, the clinical experience of many physicians using these medications in large populations fails to reveal any addictive potential.

My successful pharmacotherapy is based on the groundbreaking study of Michael Weintraub, M.D., et al. This four-year (210-week) study conducted by Weintraub, formerly associate professor of community and preventive medicine and of pharmacology at the University of Rochester School of Medicine and Dentistry, now with the Food and Drug Administration, concluded that a combination of two prescribed appetite-suppressant medications is valuable in helping obese people lose weight and maintain that weight loss. The medications—fenfluramine and phentermine—were taken daily as part of a weight-loss strategy that also included behavior modification, caloric restriction, and regular exercise.

The results of this study were reported in a series of articles in the May 1992 issue of *Clinical Pharmacology and Therapeutics*. The following is a summary of pertinent phases of the study.

Initial Phase

The study began with 121 participants between eighteen and sixty years of age who were seriously and chronically overweight, weighing on average over 54 percent over their ideal body weight as measured by the 1983 Metropolitan Life tables. The subjects were instructed in nutrition, exercise, and behavior modification and then were divided into two groups: one that took active medication and a placebo group that took capsules with no active medication. After 34 weeks, the group taking active medications—60 mg of fenfluramine and 15 mg of phentermine—lost an average of 15.9 percent of their initial weight (36 pounds, on average) compared to the 4.6-percent loss (7 pounds, on average) by the placebo group.

Continuous Dosing vs. Intermittent Dosing

Between weeks 34 and 104 of the study, different schemes were examined for administering the medications—continuously, intermittently (stopping and starting), and on an augmented basis—to both the original medicated group *and* the placebo group. Of special note: Once the placebo group began the active medications, they eventually reached the same weight-loss level as the participants in the continuously treated group.

Conclusion: Continuous medication seems superior to intermittent (stop and start) therapy due to side effects (primarily dry mouth) and some weight gain during periods without medication.

Final Phase

During weeks 190 to 210, the final phase of the study, all participants stopped taking the medications but continued to exercise regularly and eat appropriately. By the last week, most of the subjects had regained the weight they had lost.

Conclusion: Without the medication, study participants had a difficult time keeping their weight off.

Length of Treatment

Clearly, one of the major results of Weintraub's study was the confirmation of the chronicity of obesity. Also, that fenfluramine and phentermine are *safe, effective, and nonaddicting when used on a chronic basis.* Treatment must be individualized and it is important to develop a one-to-one approach with each patient and adjust medications as necessary. I use the drug combination for a three- to six-month period and then make an assessment of the patient's condition.

When evaluating a patient and before suggesting pharmacotherapy, I take into account family history, percentage of body fat, and medical conditions, such as sleep apnea disorder, diabetes, hypertension, lipid abnormalities, and musculoskeletal disorders such as back problems.

I recommend starting patients on phentermine and fenfluramine if they are not pregnant or contemplating pregnancy and if they have no medical contraindications, such as unstable cardiac conditions, uncontrollable hypertension, serious psychiatric disorders, use of MAOI medication, alcoholism, or a history of drug abuse. Patients may need to have their hypertension treated with medication prior to initiating phentermine and fenfluramine therapy. Any psychiatric problems that are primary or the result of the obesity need to be effectively treated. I frequently prescribe antidepressants in combination with the anti-obesity drugs.

Phentermine is a mild stimulant, so it's best to use the medications in the morning to reduce risk of sleep problems. I typically start with 15 mg of phentermine taken before 10 A.M. Fenfluramine, a mild depressant, can conveniently be used in the evening. I prescribe 20 mg of fenfluramine to be taken around 4 P.M. or 5 P.M.

The most common side effect of the medications is dry mouth. Other side effects reported include abdominal pain, nausea, metallic taste, diarrhea, and constipation.

I do not alter the dosage for two to four weeks. This allows time for the patient to adjust to the medications. If the patient requires additional medication, I will add an additional 20 mg of fenfluramine to the regimen. This second dose can be taken either with the morning phentermine dose or between noon and 1 P.M. Very rarely, I will have to increase the dose of phentermine to 30 mg in the morning. The lowest dose of the medications that results in weight loss, with decreased appetite, is the dose I would use for daily maintenance. You can expect a 15-percent to 20-percent reduction of body weight in almost all of your patients.

I usually continue the medications for three to six months, at which point I attempt to reduce and eventually eliminate them. I am clear in my instructions to the patient. Should the patient start to regain some weight—more than 10 pounds—the medications should be restarted and taken for a variable period of time.

In addition to the medications, it is clear that appropriate low-fat, lower-caloric eating programs are suggested. Moreover, an exercise program that is guided by a fitness evaluation suggests that exercise sufficient to improve fitness and muscle strength is essential for every patient.

For any physician interested in managing patients with weight problems, I would strongly suggest reading *Obesity*, by

Stunkard et al. (Raven Press, 1993) and *Treatment of the Seriously Obese Patient,* by Wadden and VanItallie (Guilford Press, 1992).

I have found long-term pharmacotherapy to be an effective, well-tolerated, and safe tool in the management of obesity. I would be delighted to hear your comments and experiences.

Respectfully,
Steven Lamm, M.D.
Clinical Assistant Professor of Medicine
New York University Medical Center

References

1. Weintraub M, Sundaresan PR, et al. Long-term weight control study. *Clin. Pharmacol. Ther.* 1992; May 51(5):586–646.

2. Bray GA. Barriers to the treatment of obesity. *Ann. Intern. Med.* 1991; 115:152–3.

3. Silverstone JT. Appetite-suppressant drugs. In Stunkard AJ, Wadden TA, eds. *Obesity: Theory and Therapy,* 2nd ed. New York: Raven Press, 1993, 275–85.

4. Tuominen S, Hietula M, Kuusankoski M. Double-blind trial comparing fenfluramine, phentermine and dietary advice on treatment of obesity. *Int. J. Obes.* 1990; 14 (Suppl 2):138.

5. Guy-Grand B, Apfelbaum M, Crepaldi G, Gries A, Lefebvre P. International trial of long-term dexfenfluramine in obesity. *Lancet* 1989; 2:1142–5.

6. Turner P. Dexfenfluramine: Its place in weight control. *Drugs.* 1990; 39 (Suppl 3):53–62.

7. Leibowitz SF. Neurochemical-neuroendocrine systems in the brain controlling macronutrient intake and metabolism. *Trends in Neuroscience.* 1992; 15:491–7.

8. VanItallie TB. Metabolism: Introduction. *Metabolism.* 1995; 44, No 2 (Suppl 2):1–3.

9. *Weighing the Options: Criteria for Evaluating Weight-Management Programs.* Washington, D.C.: National Academy Press, 1995.

10. Abenhaim L, Moride Y, et al. Appetite-Suppressant Drugs and the Risk of Primary Pulmonary Hypertension. *N. E. J. Med.* August 29, 1996; 335, No. 9.

11. Manson, JE, Faich, GA. Pharmacotherapy for Obesity—Do the Benefits Outweigh the Risks? *N. E. J. Med.* August 29, 1996; 335, No. 9.

Acknowledgments

Writing a book is an endeavor supported, helped, and nurtured by many people. First and foremost, to Nancy and Herb Katz, our literary agents, our deepest appreciation and gratitude. Your initial enthusiasm, skill, and insistence that this book become the best it could be so ably guided us from the first planning stages straight through the final review process. Your contributions have been innumerable and outstanding.

Our heartfelt thanks to Jean Arbeiter for her thoughtful attention and invaluable contributions to the reviewing and shaping of the manuscript. We would also like to thank Nathan Rosen, a true professional who provided us with his research assistance.

Our warm thanks to Barry Zide, M.D., and Frank Michel for their candor, wit, and astute observations in the preparation of the manuscript. Our gratitude also is extended to several friends and colleagues who took time from their busy schedules to read the manuscript and offer helpful comments and advice: Michael Margulies, Susan Taman Levy, and Donna Couzens. Thanks also to Charles Kaner, D.D.S., for his insight and experience in this subject matter and his overwhelming support for our position. And, of course, special thanks to Jack Simpson, for his extraordinary sense of style and grace.

Special thanks and appreciation to our editor, Fred Hills, for his invaluable suggestions and keen understanding of our purpose; and thanks as well to Carolyn Reidy and Michele Martin, who believed in the importance of our message from the outset. And we would be remiss if we did not acknowledge the fine assistance of Hilary Black.

We are also grateful to the following physicians and scientists for their help with various parts of the book: Michael Weintraub, M.D., Glenn Braunstein, M.D., G. Michael Steelman, M.D., Barry Jacobs, Ph.D., Sarah Leibowitz, Ph.D., and Bobby Sandage, Ph.D. James Merker and William Boni provided key contacts, and for their kind direction, we are thankful.

We would also like to gratefully acknowledge Dr. Lamm's patients, from whom we have learned so much and whose experiences are the very foundation of this book. You so willingly agreed to be extensively interviewed and you detailed so much of your lifelong struggles with weight. The publication of this book has been inspired by your desire to take charge and achieve maximum well-being in your life. Without you, this book never would have been published.

Steven Lamm, M.D., and Gerald Secor Couzens
New York, N.Y.

Index

weight loss (*cont.*)
  metabolic changes and, 144–45,
    183
  sagging skin and, 200–01
  speed of, 192, 197, 198–99
  variables in, 198–99
  in Weintraub study, 52–55
  see also specific topics
weights, making, 222
Weight Watchers, 41, 77
Weintraub, Michael, 24, 36, 44–45,
    48–57, 78
  fenfluramine-phentermine
    research of, 49–57, 66, 159, 162,
    197, 238–39

white fat, 186
wind trainers, 219
women:
  resistance training for, 132–35,
    205
  unrealistic weight standards of, 12,
    14–15, 21
workout partners, 137

Xenical, 185

yo-yo dieting, psychological dangers
  of, 20–21, 143

Zoloft, 201

About the Authors

Steven Lamm, M.D., is an internist and assistant clinical professor of medicine at the New York University School of Medicine. He received his undergraduate training at Columbia University, and his medical degree and clinical training at New York University School of Medicine. He is a member of the Presidents' Commission on University Health Matters, the New York State Athletic Commission, as well as Alpha Omega Alpha (the honor medical society), and the American Medical Association. Dr. Lamm is a regular guest on New York network television news programs, offering his analyses and comments on a wide variety of health and medical-related topics, and is frequently quoted in *The New York Times*. He is also a consultant to *American Health* magazine. He lives in New York City.

Gerald Secor Couzens is the former syndicated fitness columnist for New York *Newsday*. He writes about fitness and health issues for various publications, and is a contributor to the *University of California at Berkeley Wellness Reports*. He lives in New York City.

WE'D LOVE TO HEAR FROM YOU!

We're eager to know:

- How you heard about *Thinner at Last*. Did a friend recommend it? Did your doctor suggest it? Or did you learn about it on the Internet, or via some other medium?

- How *Thinner at Last* is different from other weight-loss books you've read.

- Whether the tear-out section for your physician was well received.

- If you would like to receive a *Thinner at Last* newsletter. (If so, please be sure to include your name and address in your correspondence to us.)

Thank you for your time and effort.

Be well,

Steven Lamm, M.D.
Thinner at Last
P.O. Box 50090
Provo, Utah 84605-0090